Dr Susan Albers is a clinical psychologist at the Cleveland Clinic. She specialises in weight loss, body image and emotional eating. She blogs for *Psychology Today, More* and the *Huffington Post* and is regularly interviewed for *O, the Oprah Magazine, Women's Health, Prevention, Family Circle* and the *Wall Street Journal.*

Praise for *Quit Comfort Eating*:

'If you want to lose weight you need to change your relationship to food. This book is a great place to start' Danny Penman, co-author of *Mindfulness: A practical guide to finding peace in a frantic world*

'At last – a book on eating well that puts everything you need to know in one place. Brilliant!' Dr Christiane Northrup

'Dr Albers shows you how to shore up a solid emotional and mental foundation to sustain a healthy diet for years to come. If you want your healthy eating plan to last, read *Quit Comfort Eating*' Shirzad Chamine, author of *Positive Intelligence*

'The key to achieving a long-term love affair with your body (and your food!) isn't about fad diets or guilt trips to the scale. It's about harnessing your emotions. Susan's game plan to turn the proven power of emotional intelligence into eating intelligence means happier, healthier, smarter eating!' Daphne Oz, chef, bestselling author, and co-host on ABC's *The Chew*

'This book gives readers a roadmap to help them gain better understanding of why they eat what they eat' Dr Lilian Cheung, co-author of *Mindful Eating, Mindful Life* and Director of Health Promotion & Communication, Department of Nutrition, Harvard School of Public Health

'Susan Albers has done it again. *Quit Comfort Eating* is full of effective and practical tools that illuminate how we have the capacity, with our own awareness and hearts to have a wiser relationship to food and step into a life of greater nourishment, freedom and joy' Elisha Goldstein, Ph.D., author of *The Now Effect* and co-author of *A Mindfulness-Based Stress Reduction*

QUIT COMFORT EATING

LOSE WEIGHT BY MANAGING YOUR EMOTIONS

DR SUSAN ALBERS

piatkus

This book is dedicated to all those who are on their journey
toward healthy, smart, savvy eating

PIATKUS

First published in the US as *EAT.Q.* in 2013 by HarperOne,
an imprint of HarperCollins Publishers
First published in Great Britain in 2013 by Piatkus

This book is written as a source of information only. The information contained
in this book should by no means be considered a substitute for the advice of a
qualified medical professional, who should always be consulted before beginning
any new diet, exercise, or health regime.

Throughout this book, the author refers to her clients, friends and people
who have shared their stories. To protect their confidentiality, the author has
changed their names and identifying characteristics.

A CIP catalogue record for this book
is available from the British Library.

ISBN 978-0-7499-5945-6

Printed and bound by CPI Group (UK) Ltd, Croydon, CR0 4YY

Papers used by Piatkus are from well-managed forests
and other responsible sources.

MIX
Paper from
responsible sources
FSC
www.fsc.org   FSC® C104740

Piatkus
An imprint of
Little, Brown Book Group
100 Victoria Embankment
London EC4Y 0DY

An Hachette UK Company
www.hachette.co.uk

www.piatkus.co.uk

CONTENTS

FOREWORD

Want to know a secret? One of the best things you can do for your health is to eat glorious food, but not too much and not too little. You know, it's that curious and enigmatic place between two worlds that few have mastered. I've discovered in my past two decades of taking care of patients that most know *what* to eat, but they struggle with *quantity*, or they eat for *reasons other than hunger*, usually related to emotions and old dysfunctional patterns.

Not surprisingly, knowledge of *what* to eat doesn't get you very far when it comes to the sacred trip of fork to mouth.

I know about such things as a Harvard-educated integrative physician and author of the *New York Times* bestseller *The Hormone Cure*. Mostly, I know about the problems of food and weight by virtue of being human for the past four decades. In fact, I live those issues at least three times per day!

If you are similar to most people who struggle with food, whether you are overweight or not, you spend way too much of your day thinking about, romanticizing, and planning what you'll eat. Perhaps you make radical vows on most Mondays to try the latest fad diet. Maybe your ears perk up when someone you know has the latest supplement that you hope might solve, once and for all, your trouble with food. (Sadly, that supplement doesn't exist. They simply make your urine more expensive.) Even more likely, you eat when stressed. Deadlines loom, your kid is sick, your parent needs you, and there's just no time—you eat to soothe the stress hormones that are wreaking havoc in your system.

Introducing Dr. Susan Albers

That's where Dr. Susan Albers comes in. Susan is not just any psychologist: she specializes in mindful eating, mindfulness, emotional intelligence, weight loss, and, *oh yes,* the many struggles we experience around body image.

The short version: Susan is exceptional. She is the psychologist to read and be guided by. Give her permission to help you heal your rocky relationship to food. Susan wrote a powerful book, which you now hold in your hands, and it has the potential to upgrade your relationship to food and transform your life. Her new book, *Quit Comfort Eating,* is a fascinating and can't-put-it-down hybrid of emotional intelligence and how to apply it to the food on your fork.

Susan is not just the latest nutrition expert du jour. She is currently a practicing psychologist who works one-on-one with clients. Susan earned a doctorate in psychology, served her internship at the University of Notre Dame, and completed her postdoctoral work at Stanford University. She has been publishing her crucial work for a decade about how to eat mindfully, and she has improved the lives of thousands of people as she teaches them the practical tips that move the needle on food, particularly cognitive retraining and behavioral tweaks. That alone makes me want to be her client and her friend, and maybe invite her over for some kale and quinoa.

Lessons Learned from *Quit Comfort Eating*

Quit Comfort Eating has upgraded my own relationship to food and transformed my life. Honestly, Susan had me at the Venn diagram in chapter 1. She knits together the most important psychological concepts of our time and applies them to my fork. How incredible is that?

Emotional intelligence (EI) is all about how to be smarter about our connections with people. But now, Susan applies the tenets of EI to food, and that's a very good thing. In her own fun and pithy language, she points out that what works for leaders also works for eaters. Her checklists are powerful tools that illuminate everything you need to know about your eating style.

Part Road Map, Part Coach

Like most of us, you've probably heard Michael Pollan's mantra: "Eat food. Not too much. Mostly plants." While I love Michael Pollan, when he tells me not to eat too much, I suddenly feel rebellious and want to do the opposite. I channel Eve in the Garden of Eden—but instead of an apple, I'm seeking my avalanche food. Hello, peanut butter? Dark chocolate?

Susan provides the road map. And she's the best person for the job. She is besotted with untangling your problems with food and applying eating intelligence. It's devastatingly persuasive. I'm going to go out on a limb and say it's smartest book I've read on upgrading how you eat.

Who doesn't need that? In all my years taking care of women and men, I've met only a handful of naturally mindful eaters. For instance, my friend Allison slices off the tiniest little piece of cheese when our families get together for dinner. *Her slice of cheese is so thin, it's sheer. She puts it on a gluten-free cracker and takes one tiny bite.* Then she puts it down on a plate and chews mindfully, about thirty times before swallowing. She enjoys every bite without a hint of worry or the fear of overeating too many crackers. That's a *mindful eater.* They are exceedingly rare.

The rest of us need this book.

Some folks who've mastered a topic are able to make it simple yet compelling. Susan has done that in *Quit Comfort Eating.* She offers her broad and deep understanding of why we overeat despite knowing better. More important, she offers alternatives. Not insane, yeah-right alternatives, but palatable ones. The type of remedies that a friend mentions over dinner, and you lean in, riveted by her wisdom.

It's Time

Quit Comfort Eating is disarming in its simplicity. As I read Susan's book, large chunks of available time to read it properly suddenly became available—because I was so intrigued by this new way of thinking. I realized she taps into the most urgent barriers that I have to eating glorious food.

You want this. It rewires your brain for the better.

I used to think, back in my twenties, that I could make up for my caloric excesses with exercise, and then I confronted the truth in my thirties, that food is most of the equation. In fact, about 70 percent of your weight is related to the food on your fork, from its nutragenomic value (how it interacts with your genes), to how it is eaten (savored or wolfed down), to quantity.

Here's what I wish for you: peace around food. I want you to eat with intelligence. I want you to not just read this book, but put Susan's wise counsel into action today—this minute, this hour. Don't put it off, because your relationship with food just might be the most important relationship in your life. It's nearly impossible to be a loving spouse or parent or even to complete your mission if you've got a strained relationship to food.

This is her best book yet. It's smart. It's informed. It's time.

Keep reading.

—Dr. Sara Gottfried
SaraGottfriedMD.com
Berkeley, CA

PART ONE

What Is Eat.Q.?

The right time to eat is:
for a rich man when he is hungry,
for a poor man when he has something to eat.

—Mexican proverb

Some of the smartest people I know overeat. They are successful in business, responsible, and creative. They know what a healthy lifestyle looks like: more fruits and vegetables, fewer processed foods, regular exercise. Intellectually, they know they would benefit from eating healthier, yet they find they are unable to improve their diets. My clients have asked one particular question over and over: "How can I *know* how to eat well and not be able to *do* it?" They wonder why their decisions don't match the way they desire to eat. The answer to this question is complex, but it will be made clearer throughout this book. To give you a hint, more often than not it's a feeling or an emotion that lies in the gap between your decision and your actions.

When did choosing what to eat become so hard?

For a very long time in human history *deciding* to eat was a luxury. Most people scrabbled and scraped for food, and ate when it was available rather than when they wanted to. Emotional eating is a relatively new phenomenon, rooted in the recent ability to choose from an array of cheap, plentiful, pleasurable foods.

For better or worse, we have more choices than ever before. Starbucks alone boasts that it has eighty-seven thousand different drink combinations to pick from—not including their food options.

The result? We no longer eat when food is available, because it's almost always available. We eat for lots of reasons, but physical hunger—the rumble and ache of an empty stomach—is not always at the top of the list.

Today, every morsel you put in your mouth—meal or snack, diet food or comfort food, just enough or too much—begins with a decision, and each decision is rooted in a feeling. Emotional eating results from a lack of particular skills that help a person cope with the intensity and duration of his or her feelings, instead of stuffing those feelings down, numbing them out, turning them off, or escaping them with comfort foods. Unfortunately, these skills aren't taught in schools, and it's tough for caregivers to teach techniques they may not have down pat themselves. These skills—the ability to perceive, use, understand, and manage emotions—were defined as *emotional intelligence* by psychologists just a few decades ago. Even then emotional intelligence skills were used almost exclusively in the lofty worlds of business and finance. Now, in this book, I will show you how to move these same skills from the boardroom table to the kitchen table.

As a psychologist who has spent more than a decade counseling people on ways to improve their diets, I believe that without the skills linked to emotional intelligence, the urge or desire to eat—which is stoked by feelings, both positive and negative—will trump even the most valiant efforts to avoid overeating. The solution is to learn to identify what you're feeling in that critical moment of decision and to manage that feeling so you can make a healthier eating decision. And you *can* learn. I've helped people do it. I'm happy to share with you everything I know.

I'd like to welcome you to *Quit Comfort Eating*, a set of skills and strategies that develop emotional intelligence as well as *mindfulness,* the ability to pay close attention to what your feelings are telling you in the moment. Together, these skills and strategies constitute the EAT method, which enables you to Embrace your feelings, Accept your emotions, and Turn to new, positive alternatives. When you learn and practice this method, you'll take control of your eating decisions, manage your cravings, conquer emotional and stress eating, and manage your weight once and for all. As a bonus, you'll improve your relationships, boost your self-confidence, and experience eating as the pleasure it's meant to be. That's *Quit Comfort Eating* in action!

1

The Solution to Emotional Eating, Stress Eating, and Plain Old Overeating

To eat is a necessity; to eat intelligently is an art.

—La Rochefoucauld (French writer, 1613–1680)

Do you make a healthy dinner or pick up fast food? Choose a salad or fries? A doughnut or fruit? Accept a second helping or say, "No, thank you"? These are simple questions that would seem to lead to straightforward decisions. Yet choosing what to eat can be one of the toughest choices you make all day. It's rarely hunger that makes this task so daunting. Instead, emotions have

food for THOUGHT

- Are you more "book smart" or "people savvy"?
- Is there a gap between your intention to eat well and your ability to do it? If so, where do you think this gap comes from?
- Can you identify the emotions that affect your eating the most? Stress? Anxiety? Boredom? Anger? What aspect of these feelings drives you toward food?
- In what ways do you feel you may use food to change your mood? For example, do you eat to entertain yourself, put off unpleasant tasks, or avoid uncomfortable feelings (sadness, loneliness, boredom, anger)?
- Which feelings typically help you eat the right foods for you, in the right amounts for you?

an incredible power to steer food decisions in the opposite direction of your intentions—often 180 degrees away from healthy eating.

I witnessed this phenomenon in action just the other day as I worked on my laptop (on this very book!) at my favorite coffee shop in Denver. My table was only a few feet from the glass display case brimming with a dizzying array of pastries, with healthier offerings like fruit salad and Greek yogurt in front of and below the glass. I had a perfect vantage point to observe the line of customers as I wrote.

An attractive, middle-aged woman in an expensive suit, holding a designer leather briefcase, drew my attention. As she waited in line, she glanced at her watch, shifted from foot to foot impatiently, and sighed as her mobile phone beeped with multiple e-mails.

When she reached the front of the line, the woman—who mere seconds before had appeared poised and confident—looked into the pastry case and froze.

The barista waited patiently; the customer behind her continued to text, unperturbed. Only I could see the struggle in her eyes.

A good twenty seconds later—forever, when you're ordering at a popular coffee shop during the morning rush—she pointed to a large scone lavishly topped with icing. "That," she said, her voice resigned.

She took a seat at a table next to mine, and our eyes met.

"I don't know why I chose this," she said. "I'm trying to eat healthier. I could have picked up a fruit salad or a container of yogurt. I don't even really want this." She glanced down at the enormous pastry on her plate.

Though I kept my eyes on my laptop, I noticed that she ate about half the scone—plump, glistening with icing. Then she stood up, walked to the bin, and slid the other half off her plate and into its dark depths.

As I observed this woman—the encounter lasted less than five minutes—I picked up on two things. First, this woman clearly had trouble deciding what to eat. Second, I see this food-related hesitation and doubt all around me in even the smartest and most successful people. Essentially, I saw and felt, at a gut level, that choosing what to eat—and not to eat—is a decision fraught with a surprising level of difficulty and emotion.

Maybe you can relate. After all, you too face an endless stream of food choices and make literally hundreds of decisions a day about what to eat.

Every day I see clients who want to improve their eating habits. Everything about this woman—her style, bearing, manner—identified her as someone who makes countless decisions in her office each day, each one demanding that she be reasoned, rational, and logical. Nevertheless, my practiced eye had seen her come undone by a task that seems simple yet is more complex than we know: deciding what to eat.

I'd bet a cup of my favorite coffee that at the moment she'd pointed to that scone, stress had weakened her ability to make a decision in line with her goals. *Was* she stressed? Her body language—shifting her feet, sighing, checking her watch—suggested so. Maybe she was between meetings and still had to hop on a plane later that day. Maybe she was running late to an important presentation.

My speculation is based on my ten years of clinical experience. Most of my clients have told me that their ability to make decisions—typically pretty good in most circumstances—nosedives when they must decide what to eat when they are stressed out.

These clients are smart and experienced decision makers. They make hundreds of decisions every day, from the trivial (which outfit to wear) to the life changing (whether to buy a multimillion-dollar company). Therefore, their food-induced indecision is curious and frustrating. Many of my clients are interested in and quite knowledgeable about nutrition. They understand why whole grains and fruits and vegetables are best, know the toxic nature of fast food and processed foods, and wonder why their nutritional knowledge isn't enough to help them "eat smart." Research backs up my clients' experiences: while learning about nutrition is helpful and necessary, knowledge sometimes has a limited impact on actual changes in behavior.[1]

With my clients, I replay moments and situations at restaurants and in their kitchens just like the situation I witnessed in the coffee shop. We start at the beginning and pinpoint the moments when things went wrong. Routinely we find that what distinguishes a healthy decision from a regrettable one is a feeling.

How is it that our feelings get in the way? How do they sabotage our decisions? Think for a moment about how your emotions affect your choices, particularly your food choices.

- When you're angry, do you develop a case of the-hell-with-its and eat foods you regret later?

- When you're anxious or under pressure, do you eat an extra slice or two of pizza?

- When you're jealous that a friend has lost weight, do you order a salad?

- When you're happy, do you eat ice cream to celebrate?

- When you're stressed, do you just give up trying to make healthier decisions and tell yourself it's just too hard?

It's likely that one if not all of these statements sound familiar. If so, keep reading. You're about to discover that what you eat—and don't eat—says volumes about the way you feel. The good news is you can use what you learn about your emotions to make positive changes in your eating habits. You'll also learn simple, science-backed strategies that can help you prevent your emotions from railroading your decisions.

Sound good? Get ready! Together, we are beginning a journey to understand how your emotions control your fork and how to put your brain back in charge.

Introducing Eat.Q.

If the woman in the coffee shop had been a client, she would have known exactly what to do *before* she selected that scone. In that make-or-break moment at the counter, she would have used her Eat.Q. to make a discerning choice based on insight rather than impulse.

Eat.Q.? What's that?

Unlike your IQ score, Eat.Q. is not a number. It's a concept that helps you align your intellectual knowledge about food and nutrition with your emotions, so you can make food choices that support your intentions and goals. You don't always choose the healthiest foods, and this is due to how you feel at that moment. Eat.Q. improves the quality of your food decisions, no matter how you're feeling.

If you can imagine food-related decisions on a line, impulsive eating would be at one end of the spectrum and thinking through each and every bite would be at the other. Most of us fall somewhere in between, but Eat.Q. moves you closer to the side of mindful eating because it rests on a specific type of self-awareness that shapes your decisions. (I call them *insight-related decisions,* and I'll discuss them in the next chapter.)

USING YOUR EMOTIONAL "DIMMER SWITCH"

I talk a lot about the importance of managing your feelings. Emotions are fluid, unpredictable, and even messy. What does it mean to *manage* feelings, and why is it so essential to improving your relationship with food?

Think of the workplace or your own job. Whether you manage others or are managed by someone else, you understand what a manager is in the context of business. Imagine all your feelings—happiness, sadness, anger, frustration, joy—as different workers with different strengths and weaknesses. When you use emotional intelligence, or EI, you're managing those workers—getting them to do what you need them to do in a kind and respectful way.

Managing your feelings is a simple term for *emotional regulation*—the ability to understand and temper your emotions so they work for you, not against you. If you overeat high-fat, sugary foods when you're feeling bad, you're attempting to manage your feelings, but in an unhealthy way. You're snapping them off like a light switch. Modern life offers plenty of ways to "snap off" your feelings. The most common are food, drugs, and alcohol, and long hours of zoning out on the Internet or in front of the TV. Unfortunately, all of them can leave you in the dark.

Emotional regulation is like a dimmer switch: you turn the "dial" of a particular emotion to the intensity that feels right to you. For example, you can "dim" a feeling of rage to a more manageable emotion of anger or irritation.

You may already be using emotional regulation skills, including deep breathing, self-talk, journaling, and meditation. If so, great! In later chapters, you'll learn how to apply them to specific eating situations.

Because my job is to help people work through their emotions, I'm well aware of what a difficult task changing the way you eat and dealing with your feelings can be. I live and breathe it every day! That's why I'm thankful to have the opportunity to share Eat.Q. with you, as I've seen it be helpful and healing with my own clients.

The Eat.Q. model is partly based on EI because it taps into just what the woman in the coffee shop needed in that moment of choice: awareness of how she was feeling when she was deciding what to eat, a way to cope with her stress, and a strategy that would help her make a choice closer in line with what she intended.

Eat.Q. is a hybrid of three bodies of research: EI, emotional eating, and mindfulness.

- *Emotional intelligence* is a set of skills that, collectively, helps you be aware of and understand your emotions and the emotions of others, as well as how those emotions affect you and those around you. The term EI may remind you of IQ, the standard measurement of intellectual intelligence. But EI has little to do with intellectual knowledge or memorizing facts. Rather, EI taps into how well you understand your own and others' feelings, cope with stress, communicate with others, control impulses, and handle social situations. Someone with high EI may not place at the top of her class, but she's the ideal friend and coworker—personable, easygoing, doesn't easily get frustrated, and is comfortable in her own skin.

- *Emotional eating* is defined by experts as eating in response to emotions—whether positive or negative—in order to change those emotions. An example of emotional eating would be to eat to boost, numb, or soothe your mood. (*Mood* is a transient emotional state, often triggered by an event or current situation, that affects the way you process information and make decisions.)

    Thousands of research articles and books explore the complex relationship between what we feel and how we eat. But really, we've all been there. We've snacked on cookies at midnight when we can't sleep or munched mindlessly while fretting about a fight with a significant other. Eat.Q. goes beyond emotional eating to include *emotionally driven eating*, which I define as the way your current emotional state

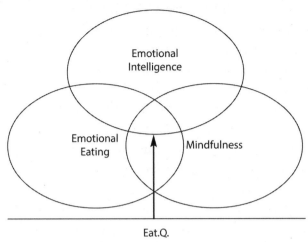

EAT.Q.

EAT.Q.

Eat.Q. is a synthesis of three concepts backed by a well-respected body of research: EI, emotional eating, and mindfulness. My clients who follow its principles, as presented in my EAT method, learn to eat better and settle at a healthier weight for the long term.

affects the quality of your food decisions. (For example, saying "I don't care what I eat" when you're angry.)

- *Mindfulness* is rooted in Buddhism. This ancient technique teaches the ability to be fully present in the moment, in a nonjudgmental way.[2] When you're mindful, you're aware of the present moment (which is not always easy when the world pulls your attention in so many different directions) and able to respond instead of react to your feelings (also not easy). Practicing mindfulness techniques can help you tune in to your feelings, which can increase your self-awareness and improve your ability to cope with uncomfortable feelings that lead you to food. In these ways, mindfulness skills can help boost your EI, often dramatically.

Let's examine the aspects of Eat.Q. In the sections that follow, I explain the theory behind each part of Eat.Q. and provide checklists, so you can see where you are right now.

Emotional Intelligence

In general, EI helps us navigate our relationships with people. Eat.Q. is the dimension of our emotional intelligence that helps us navigate our relationship with food—our overall ability to manage the relationship between what we feel and how we eat.

We all have emotions, but we experience them in different ways. For that reason, we don't deal with feelings in the same ways. Some of us are simply better at coping with feelings than others. You might be someone who is flexible and easygoing and doesn't sweat under pressure. On the other hand, you might be easily stressed out, quick to anger, or tense in uncomfortable situations. In part, these traits are innate. (Some researchers think they may be inherently part of personality.) However, coping with feelings is also a skill that can be developed and improved over time, and research suggests that it's possible to build EI.[3]

To paraphrase two pioneers of EI theory, Dr. Peter Salovey of Yale University and Dr. John D. Mayer of the University of New Hampshire, EI is the ability to accurately perceive emotions, understand their meanings, use them, and manage them in productive ways.[4] In other words, when you understand how your emotions work, you can channel them in ways that help rather than hurt you. Salovey and Mayer were among the first to explain in an organized manner why people who are very smart can find it difficult to do an ordinary task, such as communicate well with coworkers, and get frazzled over a minor issue, such as running out of printer paper.

I'm reminded of several quotes from *The Godfather* blockbuster movie series, which contains nuggets of business wisdom that hint at the tension between emotions and decision making. "It's not personal. . . . It's strictly business" is one such nugget. Another is "Keep your friends close, but your enemies closer." (This quote is actually from Sun Tzu's ancient classic *The Art of War,* but great strategists think alike!) Both sayings refer to the importance of keeping emotions in check so they don't override the ability to make beneficial decisions. It's ironic that one of the most famous lines in *The Godfather* movie involves food: "Leave the gun. Take the cannoli." Clemenza is unemotional about the killing of Paulie—completely cut off from his feelings—but doesn't want to leave the yummy cannoli behind.

A few years after Salovey and Mayer, psychologist Daniel Goleman published *Emotional Intelligence,* which sat on the *New York Times* bestseller list for eighteen months and sold more than five million copies in forty languages.[5] It became so popular in corporate America that the *Harvard Business Review* named one of Goleman's EI articles in the top ten "must-read" articles[6]. Corporations and employees began to focus on developing EI as a professional tool to increase workplace performance and results. They wanted to understand and capitalize on what makes people successful in their jobs, great leaders, and stellar employees. In the US today, other institutions, including schools and hospitals, give their employees EI training as well. Finally there was a term for why the smartest people in the world aren't always the most successful, and vice versa.

In the business world, success is defined by many things—money, recognition, power, growth—but success in business also includes concepts such as developing leadership skills, forging strong work relationships, and being resilient in hard economic times. EI isn't completely responsible for a person's success, though it does help.

But what makes a successful eater? I believe our definition has been too narrow for too long. In popular literature and magazines it has been defined in terms of weight and often with polarizing words, such as "fat" or "thin." People who are thin are even characterized as successful. (Research studies even point to this, that we hold stereotypes of people who are thin as being more attractive and successful.)[7] We assume that people who are thin are eating healthy and in perfect control of their cravings and emotions. Not so! It's time to pause and rethink how we spot a healthy eater.

Here is my proposal: stop judging who is a healthy eater based on weight and instead determine it based on his or her Eat.Q.—the quality of that person's decision-making skills around food. Successful, astute eaters, for example, can eat a sweet and then stop before they overindulge. They rarely use food to soothe themselves, or they mainly use healthy ways, such as exercise or calling a friend. They also know that at times eating is just "business" and at other times very "personal." By carefully reading the situation, they know when they should choose by the numbers (calories, fat grams, nutrients) or put their feelings first (answer a craving). They are able to choose the healthy option, even when it may not be their favorite choice. The goal is to take care of the business of the body—to feed it well and negotiate the best deal for your health and well-being.

FORGET THE DIETS—*KNOW* THYSELF!

Interestingly, both the Salovey and Mayer model and the Goleman model of EI (I admire both) highlight two specific skills: self-awareness and self-regulation. Self-awareness is the ability to look inward, to tune in to and understand your strengths, your personality traits, your quirks, how you express yourself—all the characteristics that make you tick. Self-regulation is the capacity to manage your emotions, reduce their intensity, put them into perspective, and ride them out until they fade without making them worse.

WATCH AND LEARN: EI IN ACTION

Given the choice between a salad and a cheeseburger, it's very likely that you are able to identify the healthy option. Some of you may even know the calorie count of a fast-food chain's fish sandwich versus its grilled-chicken salad, minus the croutons and cheese. So, why don't you pick the salad?

Just because you know the healthy choice doesn't mean you'll pick it, and EI skills, or lack thereof, may play a key role. Investigating the effect of teaching EI skills on food-related decision making, Paula C. Peter and David Brinberg published a study in the *Journal of Applied Social Psychology* that found when you teach people general EI skills, they make more discerning food decisions.[8] What's more, EI skills can be learned.

These are encouraging findings, because for a long time, when it came to any type of decision making, researchers viewed thoughts as separate from emotions. Now, as in this study, they're examining the interaction between the two, as well as how emotions inform the choices we make.

The first experiment of the two-part study of 120 student volunteers sought to identify EI's role in explaining why two people with the same nutritional knowledge might not make the same healthy decisions related to food, resulting in one person struggling with weight while the other does not. In it, the researchers analyzed the BMI (body mass index—a measure of body fat based on height and weight) of the students, along with their EI and both their actual (what they know) and perceived (what they think they know) nutrition and health knowledge.

For example, a boss who is self-aware and can self-regulate can recognize when she is upset. She can decide to stay in her office and cool down before leaving her desk to talk to her employees. A boss who lacks these skills may leave her office, grumble in the hallways, or snipe at people, unaware of the impact of her behavior on her employees. She may later wonder in confusion, *Why is everyone so irritable today and not working?*

The researchers found a relationship between BMI, EI, and knowledge (actual and perceived). Specifically, in students with low EI, as their knowledge increased, so did their BMIs. However, in those with high EI, as their knowledge rose, their BMIs fell. This suggests that EI skills promote the use of nutrition knowledge to benefit weight and health, and without EI, knowledge can have a negative effect on weight and health.

In the second experiment, the researchers had 146 volunteers (49 were overweight) fill out a survey of what they'd eaten in the past twenty-four hours. Then they were weighed and took part in a seventy-five-minute session of either EI training or basic information on nutrition and portion sizes. The EI training included recognizing facial expressions, understanding blends of emotions, and coping with negative feelings, such as guilt. Six weeks later, the volunteers completed the same diet survey and were weighed again. In those who were overweight, the training helped increase their ability to perceive and experience emotions and, consequently, reduce their calorie intake. Because of the study's short duration, the researchers didn't use weight gained or lost as an outcome measure; however, they hypothesized that the participants were heading in the direction of weight loss, because they were consuming fewer calories.

Based on this study's findings, it's reasonable to assume that tailoring EI skills to eating-related emotions, such as stress and anger—as the EAT method does—can actually strengthen this skill–decision connection. It worked for these students, and it can work for you too!

The skills of self-awareness and self-regulation also affect your relationship with food. When you're self-aware and can self-regulate, you quickly say to yourself, *I'm totally stressed out,* and perhaps order yourself out of the kitchen to play a computer game, knowing that it helps soothe you for the long term just as much as a bowl of ice cream. By contrast, if you typically walk into the kitchen, chomp on crisps, eat the whole bag, and then later think, *Why did I do that?* boosting your self-awareness and self-regulation skills can have a profound—and positive—impact on your eating.

While I've noticed this phenomenon with my clients, studies also suggest direct links between EI and emotional eating. To take just one example, researchers in Israel had ninety men and women aged twenty-one to sixty-two fill out questionnaires designed to examine eating attitudes and EI. They found that people with a higher EI, as measured by an EI scale, demonstrated fewer patterns of emotional eating.[9] In general, women are emotional eaters more often than men, yet even after the researchers factored in sex and age, the link between EI and emotional eating persisted.

This makes sense. If you're a person who copes well with your feelings, you're able to weigh the short-term pleasure of eating against the long-term gains to your health and emotional well-being and identify options other than eating to soothe yourself. It's the skill that determines whether you're going to be able to talk yourself skillfully through a chocolate craving or cave in to it when you're stressed out.

Please keep in mind that it's naturally harder for some people to work through their emotionally driven eating than others. In other words, some people are born with characteristics that make them prone to emotional eating and food problems. Others fall into the normal range of emotionally driven eating—it's a daily struggle, but not an insurmountable one.

WHAT WORKS FOR LEADERS, WORKS FOR EATERS

EI skills can apply to eating as easily as to business and leadership. I've constructed a chart to show just how some of the most common attributes of EI move from the boardroom table to the kitchen table. Or, for that matter, anywhere else you might be, including an office, classroom, café, four-star restaurant, or even an airplane.

EI attribute	EI in the boardroom	EI in the kitchen
Self-awareness: You know yourself well—the unique way you think, act, and feel, and how you come across to others.	You recognize your own emotions and know how they affect your thoughts and behavior at work. You've taken inventory of your strengths and weaknesses and have self-confidence that you can get the job done. You're aware of how co-workers and employees perceive and are affected by your personality.	You are tuned in to your body, your hunger level, and the way your emotions affect your decision to eat or not eat. You notice sensations and inner thoughts, such as a rumbling stomach or your mind saying *stop eating!* You know what foods you crave, your daily eating habits, and which situations or people typically derail your efforts to eat healthy. You understand how others (your significant other, friends, and children) perceive and are affected by the way you eat.
Self-regulation: You have the ability to think and calm down before you act. You're able to "dial down" strong emotions so that you remain effective.	You're able to manage and cope with your emotions in healthy ways at the office (by taking a brisk walk, meditating, calling a friend to vent) instead of taking your emotions out on others or creating negative consequences for yourself.	You use healthy mechanisms (listed in the boardroom column, or others like them) to deal with your stress level and emotions instead of working out your feelings through comfort eating. You calm down or work through your feelings before making big decisions, particularly before you open the pantry door, take another bite, or order at a restaurant.
Flexibility/ adaptation: You go with the flow.	You can handle the unexpected (a sudden meeting, a last-minute project dropped in your lap) and can adapt to an ever-changing work environment.	You can make sound eating decisions, even when there's a change in your routine. For example, if your partner wants to dine out, you're able to stick to your healthy eating plan without feeling deprived or resentful, or to choose healthy options even when you're in a new environment. You can also adjust how much you eat based on how much you ate at your last meal.

EI attribute	EI in the boardroom	EI in the kitchen
Motivation: You're driven to accomplish a goal and keep striving toward it diligently, even in the face of adversity.	For you, working hard transcends money or status; it's rooted in energy and an enthusiasm to complete a goal. You're driven by internal rewards, such as satisfaction, pride, and accomplishment of a goal.	When it comes to eating healthier, you focus on the long-term benefits to health and self-esteem rather than living or dying by a daily weigh-in. You're running a marathon, not a sprint; feeling good on the inside and improving your self-esteem and confidence (rather than a number on the scale) keeps you on track.
Empathy: You're able to put yourself in someone else's shoes.	You possess a strong awareness of other people's needs, concerns, and feelings, along with the ability to understand and respond to other people's emotions. You communicate in a way that shows you understand how your employees and coworkers feel.	You're compassionate and understanding of your own and other people's struggles with food. Empathy gives you a nonjudgmental attitude, which counters critical, self-sabotaging thoughts that talk you out of eating well.
Optimism: You have a positive outlook.	You can continue to be hopeful despite adverse conditions or setbacks on the job.	You can be positive about changing your eating habits. You stay encouraged and work through feelings of guilt or errors when you overeat. Most important, you know that adapting your eating habits for the better is possible—you retain hope even when you feel frustrated.
Impulse control: You can resist temptation for an immediate reward and wait for a later reward.	You can be patient and exercise self-control and willpower. You can hold off on a deal now with the knowledge that a	You're able to exercise self-control around pleasurable foods. You can forgo the immediate reward of a tasty treat (even when you really want it!) for the long-term, future

EI attribute	EI in the boardroom	EI in the kitchen
Impulse control: (continued)	more lucrative or rewarding offering may come in the future.	benefits of managing your weight and improving your health.
Social skills: You have the ability to work well and communicate with others.	You have the ability to build rapport and find common ground with others, and to communicate, persuade, and lead change. For example, you can tactfully give feedback to employees or say no to a request in a way they understand and appreciate.	You're able to negotiate your needs with the needs of others (what you want to eat versus what your significant other or children want to eat). You skillfully handle social eating situations, such as holiday parties and dining out, without overindulging. You're able to say no to food pushers in a skillful and tactful way and eat with other people without caving in to the pressure to mimic the ways they eat.

Now that you've been introduced to some of the most beneficial EI skills, perhaps you're wondering about your own EI skills. In the checklist that follows, see which characteristics of EI you already have that will serve you well in the kitchen!

CHECKLIST: EI SKILLS

This checklist* is based on the characteristics common among high-EI people. Some statements focus on how well you perceive your own feelings, some pertain to reading other people, and some focus on coping with and monitoring your reaction to difficult feelings. Check all the statements that apply to you.

*For a formal assessment, consider taking the Mayer-Salovey-Caruso Emotional Intelligence Test (MSCEIT). For more information on this test, including how to take it, visit mhs.com.

▶

Know, however, that we all have areas of EI that are stronger than others. For example, maybe you intuitively understand and are able to cope with other people's feelings but have difficulty identifying and expressing your own. No matter what your challenges, you're sure to have some strengths on which to build. This simple tool can help you start to think about them and zero in on your challenges.

____ I know what I'm feeling as I feel it.

____ I can typically zero in on *exactly* how I feel. (For example, rather than "upset," you use specific words like "angry" or "frustrated.")

____ I'm good at putting how I feel into words.

____ I feel empathy for other people.

____ I make a decision quickly and/or easily.

____ I'm flexible and can go with the flow.

____ I think about what I'm feeling and try to understand why I feel the way I do.

____ I learn from past experiences and don't often repeat the same mistakes.

____ I'm a good judge of character, mostly.

____ I generally don't get too stressed out, and I have healthy ways of dealing with stress.

____ I'm optimistic that things will work out.

____ When a friend is upset, I help talk him or her through it. Strong emotions or tears don't upset me.

____ I'm okay with confronting issues head-on.

____ If I make mistakes, I know this is human and I try not to criticize or beat myself up over it.

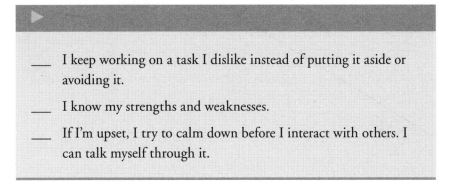

> ___ I keep working on a task I dislike instead of putting it aside or avoiding it.
>
> ___ I know my strengths and weaknesses.
>
> ___ If I'm upset, I try to calm down before I interact with others. I can talk myself through it.

Did you find that you already have many strong EI skills? Great! Before long, you'll know how to transfer these skills over to specific eating situations, such as how to stop picking at your plate even though you're full or how to stop overeating cookies just because they taste so good.

Emotional Eating

When I'm stressed, I stuff myself with chocolate.

When I'm bored, I mindlessly munch on crisps and dip until I polish off a bag.

After a very long, frustrating day, a bowl of ice cream calms me instantly.

If you identify as an emotional eater, these statements probably ring true. But what if you eat comfort food not because you want to soothe stress or relieve boredom, but because when you're in a bad mood, you don't care what you choose?

Emotions, both positive and negative, steer our thoughts and choices. In this book, I use the term *emotionally driven eating* in place of *emotional eating*. That's because while not everyone is an emotional eater, everyone's decisions are affected by his or her emotions.

Have you ever been on one of those amusement-park rides that spin so quickly its riders are pushed against the wall? As the floor drops out, riders "stick" to the wall thanks to centrifugal force, a force created by circular motion that pushes you away from the center. Emotions are much like centrifugal force—they can spin you so quickly that you get pushed away from your true center, the direction you intended.

Emotional eating is a consumptive response to emotions. If you become stressed at work, you eat. If you break up with your partner, you eat. Often emotions you're not conscious of lurk behind unhealthy food decisions and overeating. Consciously or unconsciously, you choose food in an attempt to change your emotional state—to boost your mood, ease your pain, relieve your stress.

With emotionally driven eating, your choices are based, in part, on how you feel at the moment you decide if, what, when, and how much you're going to eat. Maybe you've heard yourself say, "I'm too stressed out. I can't start eating healthy right now." *That's* emotionally driven eating. Similarly, your decision to stuff down a brownie depends, in part, on whether you feel relaxed or stressed. Many of my clients tell me that when they're in the grips of negative emotions, such as anger, sadness, or stress, their feelings outweigh the other aspects important to the decision-making process (taste, nutritional quality, visual appeal, the likelihood of feeling regret). On a calmer day, they can think through all the information before making a choice. The bottom line is that feelings and thoughts influence your actions.

One of my clients, Jill, recently gave me an example of an emotionally driven decision. She was meeting a friend, Janet, for lunch. Jill arrived first, perused the menu, and decided on fried chicken, a dish she loves but doesn't make at home. Then Janet walked in, looking fit and gorgeous.

"I was jealous," Jill told me, and that envy changed her choice. While Janet didn't *want* a salad, her mood shifted when she saw her friend, and her feelings influenced her choice. (Alas, sometimes you don't pick the healthier option. You might pick the double cheeseburger instead of the salad.)

Emotionally driven decisions can also arise from positive feelings. For example, spaghetti sauce boiling on the stove may remind you of your grandmother, who often urged you to eat seconds of her pasta. The warmth of that memory may drive you to eat, even though you aren't really hungry. Or maybe you order a particular kind of bow tie pasta salad with olives because it reminds you of your first love—that is what he would have ordered.

The good news is that Eat.Q. can help both emotionally driven eating and emotional eating. The goal is to become aware of and understand the mood–food connection instead of cutting it off.

CHECKLIST: EMOTIONAL EATING OR EMOTIONALLY DRIVEN EATING

You may be wondering if you're vulnerable to emotional eating or emotionally driven eating. Put a check mark by the statements that apply to you.

____ When overwhelmed, I think, *What the heck. I might as well eat what I want.*

____ I tend to make better food decisions in the morning, when I'm fresh, and the worst decisions at night, when I'm tired and unwinding.

____ When I'm stressed, I just don't care what I eat.

____ I'm vulnerable to emotional eating—calming and comforting myself with food.

____ When I celebrate, I use eating to conjure up the spirit of the occasion. (For example, if I'm on holiday, I should eat whatever I want.)

____ I entertain myself with food when I'm bored.

____ Munching on food distracts me from what I'm feeling.

____ What people might say or think about my food choices sways my food decisions.

____ Sometimes I eat well, in the way I want, and other times I seem to have no strategy at all.

____ I tend to give up on healthy eating goals when I'm busy, waiting until the timing feels right to start eating well or after a particular event has passed.

Mindfulness

I became interested in mindfulness many years ago when I stumbled upon the concept during my studies in Japan. I also read the bestseller *Full Catastrophe Living* by Dr. Jon Kabat-Zinn, founding director of the Stress Reduction Clinic and the Center for Mindfulness in Medicine, Health Care, and Society at the University of Massachusetts Medical School. He was instrumental in bringing mindfulness into clinical research and teaching the skills in a way people could understand them and apply them to their lives. Over the past fifteen years, I've written five books and numerous articles about mindful eating, and I use mindfulness in my own life and in my work with clients.

Many of our food choices, for better or worse, are mindless habits that develop into routines—choosing the same cereal day after day, ordering a favorite dish at a restaurant without picking up the menu. We choose what we've always chosen without really being aware of all the options. Mindfulness turns off autopilot behavior and turns on awareness, which helps people make sound decisions. With mindfulness, choices are conscious and based on awareness of what you're feeling and thinking, rather than unconscious choices based solely on habits.

Even very early in my career, I knew that emotional eaters and people with eating issues often fall into mindless habits, experience problems coping with their feelings, and use food to numb them. They are also very hard on themselves! Many of my clients have found that the nonjudgmental aspect of mindfulness has changed their lives. When they learned how to really listen to their thoughts, they realized how critical and self-sabotaging their thinking could be. You can imagine how thoughts like *How dumb could you be for eating that much!* severely affect the quality of their future decisions. Mindfulness helps you turn that negative thinking around and become more compassionate and gentle with yourself, which paves a path toward making more discerning decisions.

Like EI, mindfulness points to the idea that self-awareness and the ability to regulate feelings can help you cope with many kinds of physical and emotional pain. In other words, both EI and mindfulness are concrete skills for coping with the reality that life is hard and stressful and can lead to suffering. If you've tried to change your eating habits, you know firsthand that weight issues can be painful.

Mindfulness is stellar at helping people regulate and cope with urges, cravings, and tough emotions, and teaching it is intensely rewarding. The exercises can be pleasurable—my clients and I might eat a single slice of orange or one chocolate, savoring each sensation in the moment, or meditate, eyes closed, to soothing music. At times, the exercises are more challenging, as when I ask them to "just sit" with difficult feelings, such as sadness or disappointment, until they pass. (More often than not, they do.) Whatever the exercise, I know that, with practice, my clients will become more aware of what they're feeling in the moment—physically and emotionally—which will help them become more aware of how their feelings affect their eating decisions.

Being mindful is a way to boost your EI. To find out if you're mindful now or still a work in progress, fill out the Mindfulness skills checklist overleaf. You may notice that while many of these skills are similar to those of EI, they are unique in that they are internally focused and happening *now*, not in the past or what you anticipate about yourself in the future. You'll learn more about mindfulness skills throughout the book.

At this point, you might be wondering where your Eat.Q. stands. Is it high or low? Are you an expert or a novice? If you picked up this book, it's likely that you're still working on tweaking your skills. The checklist of Eat.Q. Skills on page 27 will give you an idea of your Eat.Q. level.

Mary: Putting the Pieces Together

In part, Eat.Q. is due to the many brave and hardworking clients I've counseled over the years. Yet it was a brilliant young woman named Mary who got the Eat.Q. concept simmering in my brain. Our work together was my first glimpse of the chasm between emotional eaters' desire to make healthy eating decisions and their painful inability to do so.

Toward the end of university, when I was working with students with eating issues at two academic institutions that accept only the brightest and most talented students, Mary came to me for help with her overeating. She was an exceptional young woman—bright, musically talented, studious, hoping to become a professor of mathematics. To her, math was reassuringly concrete—if you worked hard enough and played with the numbers, you'd find the right answer. She assumed the same was true for weight loss.

CHECKLIST: MINDFULNESS SKILLS

Place a check mark next to the skills that sound like you.

_____ I have a feeling, and I am able to recognize it right away.

_____ I think before I act.

_____ If I have an uncomfortable feeling, I can just notice it without doing anything about it.

_____ I can accept things as they are without wishing to change them.

_____ I am nonjudgmental of myself and others.

_____ I live in the moment, instead of dwelling on the past or wishing for the future.

_____ I catch myself when I slip into autopilot.

_____ I tune in to my body and my senses when I eat, noting colors, aromas, and sounds.

_____ I try to enjoy the moment without rushing through things.

_____ I really listen when people are talking to me, instead of thinking about something else.

So, at our first session Mary took a seat, gave me perfect, textbook explanations of weight loss and the principles of good nutrition, and told me what she needed: a food plan.

Even as a new psychologist with little clinical experience, I knew that while emotional eaters can follow a food plan when they feel "good," their good intentions are useless when their feelings take over their decisions.

So, instead of granting Mary her request, I gently asked if she'd be willing to record everything she ate for two weeks, along with the time, situation, and how she was feeling when she ate. Reluctantly, she agreed.

CHECKLIST OF EAT.Q. SKILLS

Put a check mark by the statements that apply to you.

____ I can identify specific feelings that typically prompt me to eat, such as boredom or stress.

____ I can identify feelings that make me lose my appetite, such as anxiety or guilt.

____ I can express my feelings to others clearly.

____ I can be flexible when plans change.

____ I can recover from an eating mistake and get back on track.

____ I'm aware of how emotions affect my decision to eat or not eat.

____ I'm empathetic toward my own and others' struggles with weight and eating issues.

____ I can distinguish between emotional and physical hunger.

____ I can listen to my body's cues (to stop eating when full, to eat for energy, and so forth).

____ I can decline food tactfully and respectfully when people urge me to eat when I'm not hungry.

____ I don't use food to avoid my feelings.

____ I can cope with uncomfortable feelings.

____ I'm flexible in thinking about food.

____ I'm attuned to my own eating and don't consciously, or unconsciously, mimic the way other people eat.

____ I can cope with stress without it having a negative impact on my eating decisions.

____ I can respond effectively to a craving, either answering it without eating too much or letting it go.

Two weeks later, her entries revealed a pattern: the day before a stressful event, such as an exam or a violin recital, she went off the plan and back to her old ways of eating (lots of high-fat snacks and late-night sweets). For Mary, reluctant to talk or even think about her feelings, this simple observation was a milestone. For the first time she could *see* the connection between what she ate and how she felt. How she felt, all the time, was afraid. She felt like an impostor, playing a brilliant student but fooling everyone, undeserving of her success and fearful of losing it.

Encouraged by her discovery, Mary continued her journal as together we took the next steps: to identify those intensely negative feelings in the moment, *as she was feeling them,* and to soothe herself enough to make a positive eating decision. These steps took more work, patience, and practice.

During this process, Mary began to see that she'd tried to reduce her eating and weight—her life itself—to a series of equations. More important, she was beginning to see why. She'd grown up with a bipolar mother who, in her manic phases, would berate her and point out her "flaws"—she was lazy, her grades weren't perfect, she wasn't a musical genius. When her mother cycled into depression, she'd lie on the sofa and ignore her daughter.

Her mother's volatile behavior incited Mary's terror, self-criticisms, and shame. To avoid her mother, and those painful feelings, Mary spent as much time at school as she could. Math was predictable, a soothing alternative to her chaotic home life, and since she always got the "right" answer no one could dispute her gift.

More and more, Mary developed her ability to identify the feelings that pushed her toward food and to manage those feelings in the moment. We also uncovered situations that triggered her urge to eat—standing in front of the overflowing buffet tables in the canteen was a big one—and devised ways to cope with them. As she learned these skills, Mary was free to decide what to eat based not on her feelings in the moment but on her *understanding* of those feelings.

Being aware of and managing the painful emotions from her childhood took diligence and persistent practice. But by the end of our work together, more often than not Mary was making healthy eating decisions and losing weight.

Mary's story reminds me of the movie *Good Will Hunting,* whose main character, Will Hunting (played by Matt Damon), has a genius-level IQ but works as a janitor at MIT. Haunted by his childhood bullying, Will is unable to use his intellect, control his temper, obtain a job that utilizes his incredible math abilities, or sustain a romantic relationship. A compassionate therapist (played by Robin Williams) helps him raise his EI skills. Gradually, through confronting, talking about, and accepting his feelings, Will increases his ability to communicate, control his impulses, and begin a serious relationship.

Mary and Will are examples of people at the extreme end of the spectrum, scoring high on IQ charts and low on EI due to past emotional abuse. However, to have low EI it's not necessary to fall at the end of the spectrum or have experienced abuse. *Everyone* can be tripped up by emotions, regardless of background or IQ. I include these examples because they illustrate well the point that EI and IQ aren't always in perfect sync.

I hope that Mary's story inspires you. It does me. Whenever a client says, "I want to change my eating, but I can't seem to do it," I think of Mary and how I can help that person boost his or her Eat.Q. in the same way.

A Road Map to This Book

Until now you could increase your ability to cope with cravings and manage your feelings primarily with one-on-one counseling, online support groups for weight loss or overeating, and workshops that teach emotion-regulation skills. Now, using the skills and tools in this book— the same ones I teach my clients—you can begin to learn how to conquer emotional or stress eating on your own. (If you have been diagnosed with or suspect you have an eating disorder, such as anorexia, bulimia, or binge-eating disorder, *please* make an appointment with a qualified doctor, psychologist, or registered dietitian who specializes in eating disorders. This book may be a step in the right direction, but it is *not* therapy.)

One thing before we begin: we won't discuss what you should eat or how much. When you're making food selections based on EI, it's not about the food. In fact, the more a client and I talk about food in our sessions, the less on track we are. A dietitian can help you choose what to eat. Our job is to raise your EI to where it needs to be, so you can identify and explore the feelings that lie beneath your eating patterns, cravings, and food choices.

In chapter 2, you'll learn the key to raising your Eat.Q.: the capacity to take a mindful pause—just long enough to make a healthy decision, rather than an emotionally driven one—and how to make a decision that serves you best. You'll also learn some core tools to help you make a sound decision at the moment it counts.

Chapter 3 outlines the EAT method. Its success depends on your ability to utilize the skills in chapter 2 and deploy tools designed to help you manage your feelings and your eating. I use them with my clients, and they're powerfully effective.

In part 2, you'll explore common barriers to raising Eat.Q.: dieting, pleasure seeking, social eating, stress, and emotional trauma. Each chapter begins with a Food for Thought section, which invites you to consider whether that particular barrier may be standing in your way.

In part 3, "Tools for Success," you'll learn twenty-five tools—those I teach my clients—which are based on cutting-edge EI research. They will help you put each part of the EAT method into practice so you can manage your eating.

As tempting as it might be to jump right in and get to work, it's important to read parts 1 and 2 before you begin part 3. Parts 1 and 2 give you an understanding of the theory and research behind Eat.Q. and the EAT method, allowing you to make the best use of the tools in part 3. *Practice* is a key word. Part 3 gives you the tools, but like muscles, they require exercise, repetition, and frequent use.

To help you practice, and to get you thinking about how your emotions affect your food choices, I've included quizzes throughout the book. They're not clinical or validated research tools, and they aren't meant to be. Rather, they're a starting point for your self-discovery. Quizzes encourage people to look inward and ask themselves questions about how they really feel and think, which helps boost their self-awareness. I hope you have fun with them and share the quizzes with others.

It's also important for you to understand that many factors play a role in healthy eating—biology, gender, access to food, and environment, to name just a few. To address them all is beyond the scope of this book. So, as you read keep in mind that this book focuses primarily on emotions, an overlooked but critical aspect of the decision-making process.

I can't promise that you'll always manage every feeling or always make the eating decision that benefits your health and well-being. But as you learn more about the emotions that drive you to seek comfort in food and sometimes sabotage your decisions, I hope you'll feel an incredible transformation and awareness grow within you. You'll be able to move ten steps ahead of and actually stop emotional eating in its tracks—now, not after the fact.

The Last Bite

Now you're ready to learn how to make smart food decisions that help rather than hinder your long-term health and weight goals. That is a big step.

In the next chapter, we'll learn about how your emotions affect your decision making.

2

The Moment of Decision

Four Tools That Instantly Boost Eat.Q.

Keep calm and carry on.

—public poster issued by the United Kingdom's
Ministry of Information, 1939

This quotation is a favorite of mine, because it so aptly describes what we all must do each day: remain calm in the midst of our stressful lives and make decisions on the fly, often under less-than-ideal circumstances.

I bought the poster just before I graduated—how perfect for a psychologist's wall, I thought.

food for THOUGHT

- What did you last "decide" to eat? How did your feelings influence your choice (were you angry at a partner, stressed at work, alone and bored, etc.)?
- Are there particular situations in which emotional eating has felt inevitable to you?
- Do you try to use logic and reason to combat cravings? If so, how successful are you?
- When you approach your refrigerator, describe your thought process as you open the door. Do you grab the first thing or contemplate at length?
- Currently, what are the best strategies you have for helping you stay calm (deep breathing, a phone call to a friend, etc.)?

How right I was. And the funny thing is that it helped me as much as my clients. Once on the job, there were many times I glanced at that poster as I worked with distraught and traumatized clients.

Unfortunately, after a few years, it was stolen right off my office wall in the middle of the night. Outraged at first, I eventually savored the irony of the situation: whoever stole it needed it far more than I! But the image and quote are forever burned into my consciousness, reminding me to try to remain unruffled as I move through my days (and nights).

Most of us have the "carry on" part down. What other choice do we have when the boiler breaks down, the bills get deep, or jobs or relationships turn rocky? It's the keeping calm part that can be a challenge. But being calm helps us make the best decisions, whether about the boiler or french fries.

The ability to keep calm requires two actions on your part. The first is psychological: being able to assure yourself that you can handle the situation, whatever it is. The second is physiological: knowing how to prevent your body from shifting into the fight-or-flight response, the primitive, inborn response that kicks in automatically when you're faced with what you perceive as a threat to your physical survival.

You'll learn more about the fight-or-flight response in chapter 7. For now, all you need to know is that when it kicks in, you're literally unable to make a decision. That's because you're too focused on survival to sift through your thoughts and feelings, which is what making a decision requires.

Our inborn *react* mode goes back millions of years, when human survival depended on making a snap decision based on instinct—to immediately turn and run in the face of immediate danger rather than weigh the pros and cons of running. (Instinct is a hardwired biological response. By contrast, intuition is rooted in a higher-level thought process.)

The fight-or-flight response is hardwired into our bodies. Today, we rarely need it—we face few immediate threats to our survival—but chronic stress and intense emotion can trigger it. The good news is you can learn to move your body and mind into a place of calm. Even better, keeping calm helps you make sound eating decisions and say no to emotional eating.

Smart decisions are neither devoid of emotion nor overshadowed or driven by it. Thus, any time you experience an emotion that typically drives you to food—be it overwhelming stress, red-hot fury, heart-wrenching sadness, or even the joy of a celebration or get-together—it's helpful to first be aware that you're feeling it, and then take steps to make decisions about eating that empower rather than derail you. And that rests on keeping calm.

Decisions, Decisions: Not Always Rational

Star Trek's Dr. Spock didn't let his emotions control or influence his thinking. If we could all make decisions as dispassionately as he, we could turn down a second slice of cheesecake when we're full without that frustrating internal tug of war between *I want* and *I shouldn't*.

However, research confirms what so many of us already know: decision making isn't always rational. Emotions are actually crucial to the brain's ability to select a course of action;[1] they're necessary to help you make decisions as minor as what to make for dinner and as life-altering as whom to marry. If you didn't factor at least some emotion into the decisions you make, it's possible you'd get caught in an endless battle of pros and cons between your options. Sometimes only a gut response can break the tie.

Although emotions influence decisions, they're not universally helpful in the process. Think of the fight with your partner when you screamed, yelled, and skipped dinner. Or the job interview you feared going to because you'd recently gained five pounds. Or that bag of crisps you demolished after a stressful day and little sleep. Understanding how your emotions affect your decision making around food can help you sort through the lure of unhealthy behaviors you know are unhealthy for you and steer you toward the actions you want to cultivate.

Thanks to our culture, eating is one of the most emotionally fraught decisions it seems a person can make. If you've been at a restaurant in a group of otherwise well-adjusted women, it's likely you heard exclamations of guilt for not ordering a salad, for ordering dessert, or for not immediately heading to the gym to burn off every single calorie. Not surprisingly, our feelings of guilt have a dramatic impact on how we decide what—and how much—to eat. Some diet foods advertise that you can eat more with none of the guilt. Linking food with emotions is potent, and advertisers know this and use it to their advantage (such as using words like "happy" and "bliss" to describe chocolate).

Different emotions affect you in various ways. Some emotions, such as anger and irritability, may prod you into making a rash decision; others, such as anxiety, stress, and fear, may leave you paralyzed, unable to decide on anything. Hundreds if not thousands of studies highlight the connection between food and feeling. (The chart below lists but a few.)

However, the research is conflicting. For example, some studies suggest that anxiety decreases food intake, while others say it increases it. To me, this contradiction indicates that researchers are still unraveling the complex factors that play a role in how emotions are intertwined with eating habits. With my clients, I've noticed that minor anxiety, such as that caused by waiting for a phone call or taking an exam, seems to lead to increases in eating. Chronic anxiety, perhaps prompted by a divorce or caring for someone with a chronic illness, sometimes makes people lose their appetite and drop weight without even trying. Thus, the nature, intensity, and duration of an emotion, as well as many other variables (gender, weight, whether or not you're on a diet), might determine whether your emotions aid your decision-making process or get in the way.

Keep in mind that everyone is unique. Some emotions will affect you in the ways shown in the studies listed below and some will not. What's important is that you're as convinced as I am that emotions do affect your food decisions.

The Emotion–Decision Connection

The handful of studies that follow suggests that emotions affect our decisions whether we like it or not.

Loneliness	How this emotion affects how much you eat may depend on whether or not you're trying to reduce your food intake, according to a study by Canadian researchers. The researchers asked fifty-eight undergraduate women to complete scientific questionnaires that assessed loneliness, depression, and disordered eating habits. Then researchers primed the participants to feel sad, lonely, or neutral, after which they ate cookies, thinking they were completing a study on taste. Women who were dieting or restricting their intake ate more cookies when they were primed to feel lonely. Those who weren't dieting, however, actually ate fewer cookies in response to loneliness.[2]

Fatigue	Fatigue may weaken our ability to sift through all the information we have in order to make a wise decision, a 2010 study published in the *American Journal of Clinical Nutrition* found. When researchers restricted the sleep of twelve healthy young men for just one night, they reported significantly higher hunger before meals the following day and subsequently ate 22 percent more calories over the course of that day.[3] Sleep difficulties are also frequently reported by people who binge eat.
Happiness	Yes, a negative mood can prompt you to eat more than you want to. But so can being in a good mood, suggests a 2010 study published in the journal *Appetite*.[4] In this study, 106 women filled out scientific questionnaires that screen for both controlled and uncontrolled emotional eating styles. (Controlled eaters have effective control of their eating; uncontrolled eaters don't.) Once tested, the volunteers were placed at random into either a group that watched a clip from a funny movie, to put them in a positive mood, or a group that watched a science documentary. After the movies, the volunteers filled out questionnaires that assessed their moods, and each volunteer had a bowl of 8 cookies placed in front of him or her as they worked. Researchers found that controlled eaters in a good mood ate 3.3 fewer cookies. However, uncontrolled eaters in a good mood ate 1.7 *more* cookies.
Sadness	In a 2013 study published in *Appetite,* researchers sorted sixty female students into groups based on extreme high and low scores on questionnaires designed to assess emotional eating. The researchers induced joy or sadness with a virtual reality system that taps into emotional movie clips and music. "High" emotional eaters ate significantly more after the sad mood condition than after the joy mood condition and ate more sweet foods than salty. By contrast, "low" emotional eaters ate similar amounts after both the sad and the joy conditions.[5] Thus, if you're an emotional eater, negative feelings might make you feel more vulnerable to eating more to comfort yourself. However, it's important to note that positive feelings can also be at the root of overeating.
Depression	In a study of more than a thousand people, higher depression scores were associated with greater chocolate consumption. In fact, a depression score suggesting major depression more than doubled chocolate consumption. That's what investigators found in the 2010 study published in the *Archives of Internal Medicine*.[6] In this study 1,018 people, who scored high on

Depression (continued)	depression as determined by their scores on the Center for Epidemiologic Studies Depression Scale (CES-D), consumed about 60 percent more chocolate compared with people with lower test scores.

Now that you've read just a few of the many studies linking feelings to food intake, the next step is to discover if specific emotions push you to eat more or less. Here's a simple exercise that can help you find out:

For one week, track how your feelings affect *all* your decisions, but particularly those that involve food and eating. Jot your observations in a small notebook. Some questions to consider: Which feelings paralyze you? Make your decisions tougher? Lead to snap decisions or indecision? Break the tie between two options?

After a week, you're bound to have a new appreciation for just how powerful emotions are. The good news is, once you're aware of how feelings affect your decisions, your ability to make decisions will improve. More often than not, emotions will support rather than hinder your intentions to eat well.

The Moment of Decision: React or Respond

The average person makes more than two hundred decisions about what to eat each day, according to research conducted by Brian Wansink, Ph.D., an expert in the fields of consumer behavior and nutritional science. [7] Some of those decisions benefit your weight and health; some don't.

What separates a decision that benefits your health and well-being from one that doesn't? One big factor is what I call the *moment of decision*—the moment you open the refrigerator, study the menu, begin your order at the drive-through: the moment you decide whether or not to eat. In that moment, as with every decision you make, thinking and feeling play equally important roles.

Before you can get a handle on the role of emotion in decision making, you must know, and acknowledge, that there is a decision to be made. In fact, your first task—which you may have to undertake with food in front of you—is to make the moment of decision a conscious one. That means slowing down enough to acknowledge that you must choose either option A (eat it) or option B (don't eat it).

Making that crucial moment conscious takes practice. Many a new client has told me, after a slip, "I thought, *No! Stop!* But as I was thinking that, I was already eating!" Or "I was halfway through my bowl of ice cream before I thought about whether I'd made the right decision—or even if I'd actually *made* a decision."

This makes sense. Some research suggests that we make decisions seven seconds before we are aware of it.[8] In other words, in many cases we don't intentionally decide before we act; we reach for food out of habit. When you're in autopilot eating mode, out of touch with what you're thinking and feeling, the moment of decision can come and go before you're even aware of it.

If you're overweight, you may make decisions more impulsively, with more negative results, than people of average weight. In a Dutch study, researchers used the Iowa Gambling Task—a psychological test that simulates real-life decision making—to compare how women with a binge eating disorder make decisions compared to average- and overweight (with a BMI above 25) women.[9] The researchers also gave their volunteers questionnaires that measured the severity of binge eating, the sensitivity for punishment and reward, and self-control.

Essentially, the Iowa Gambling Task is a card game in which you catch on to the strategy as you go. The overweight and bingeing groups performed poorly on the test—they didn't learn from their mistakes—while the average-weight women did.

Moreover, in their play, the overweight women tended to make decisions that involved short-term rewards and long-term consequences. Based on this observation, the researchers suggested that overweight women might be more sensitive to immediate rewards. That is, they may experience food and pleasurable situations as more rewarding than others do.

What do these findings mean for you? If you struggle with your weight, you may make decisions quickly and lean toward short-term rewards (pleasure *now*) versus long-term consequences (weight gain). Does that sound like you?

If it does, you can change it, starting now. At your next meal or snack, look for the moment of decision. When you find it, acknowledge it. You need do nothing more than say, either silently or aloud, "I've arrived. Here is my decision point." The next step is to make a conscious decision.

The Two Types of Decisions

"I work at home," my client Dan told me. "People tell me how lucky I am, but I've gained ten pounds since I moved from my cubicle at the office to the corner of my bedroom. Every day when I get bored or tired, I hear food calling my name. I'm very aware that I have a decision to make: either wander into the kitchen and spend twenty minutes rooting in the refrigerator or pantry, or hunker down and keep working. It's a decision I agonize over all the time."

Earlier I said that effective decision making is a combination of thought and feeling. However, my client's words aptly describe what a struggle it is to decide how to respond to the emotions that drive you to eat.

Research has shown that the decisions made by people who struggle with their weight tend to be intertwined with their emotions, which makes it more likely that their decisions will be impulsive—based solely on how they feel in the moment. Studies also show that people who struggle with their eating have difficulty tolerating their feelings—which they tend to experience intensely—and want to cut them off quickly. Tolerating your feelings means you can accept them as they are, without trying to change or react to them.

But if you're not aware of your feelings, or if you turn them off or shut them down, the quality of your decisions plummets. If you're not careful, once you open that fridge, close the menu, or begin to order at the drive-through, you'll make a decision that derails rather than supports your eating goals. I call that moment DWE—*deciding while emotional*.

The best-case scenario is that you use your emotions wisely to inform and guide your food choices. In the moment of decision, you can go one of two ways:

In an *emotion-driven decision* you react, choosing what to eat and what not to eat based on how you feel in the moment rather than on rational thought. The quality of your decisions changes based on your current emotional state. For example, let's say that five minutes from now you fly into a rage (over a traffic jam, a hurtful remark your partner made, something on the news—take your pick). Overwhelmed by anger, you eat half a bag of crisps, thinking, *The hell with it!* When you make such impulsive, emotion-driven eating choices, you're DWE.

In an *insight-driven decision* you respond, letting your feelings guide rather than dominate your decision. You perceive, predict, and prepare. You understand how your emotions can sway your decisions, anticipate the possible consequences, and manage impulses in real time instead of after the fact. In the previous example, once you've raised your Eat.Q., you perceive that you're angry, understand that you tend to make poor food decisions in anger, and can prepare to manage that anger in a positive way. Thus, you meet your moment of decision emotionally equipped to make a positive choice.

THE TWO TYPES OF DECISIONS

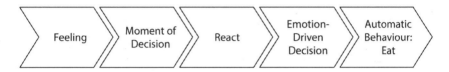

Emotion-Driven Decisions. In this model, emotions rule your food choices. At the moment you are about to make a decision, you react to your feelings automatically, which leads you to fall back on familiar behaviors.

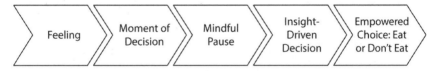

Insight-Driven Decisions. In this model, emotions influence your food choices, but as you make a food selection, you create a momentary pause to assess your intital reaction. You can fill the mindful pause with the calming tools I will share with you to help you improve the quality of your decision making.

Read the following examples of emotion- and insight-driven thinking. Which ones sound like you? Do your emotions or your insight tend to steer you toward or away from food?

Examples of emotion-driven thinking	Examples of insight-driven thinking
I want it!	If I eat that, I'll feel awful.
The hell with this diet.	I don't need this; I just want it.
It's not fair. Why can't I eat what I want?	This craving will pass.

I'm so stressed. Need. Chocolate. *Now.*	This won't help my goal to eat healthier.
This craving is too strong. I'll go crazy if I can't have pizza.	If I ate that now, I'd be soothing my feelings with food, and that never helps for more than a minute.
It's the holidays. I have to celebrate.	I can choose carefully what to eat.

The moment of decision is so pivotal. I help my clients to remember to respond, rather than react, with this reminder:

You can't decide how you feel.
You can decide what you'll eat.
Perceive, predict, prepare!

WHAT'S YOUR DECISION-MAKING STYLE?

Self-restraint (being able to manage your impulses) comes from self-awareness—both are hallmarks of emotional intelligence. Getting to know the way you make decisions can help you understand how much emotion drives your choices. Answer the following questions to gain insight into how you make decisions.

Imagine that you're holding a restaurant menu (a café, a five-star restaurant—it doesn't matter). Visualize opening it. Are you more likely to

1. choose the first item that appeals to you, and then close the menu without reading the rest of the options?

2. be plagued with indecision and have a hard time choosing an option?

3. scan the menu several times, pondering all your options, weighing the pros and cons?

4. decide spontaneously, choosing the first thing that sounds good at that moment?

5. make someone else choose because the options overwhelm you?

6. play it safe, going for what sounds the most familiar and simple?

7. order what your diet advises or what you feel you "should" have, even if it isn't what you really want?

8. skip dining out altogether because you don't want to decide?

9. tell yourself you're too busy to decide and tell the server to bring you whatever?

10. skip reading the menu and choose based on what looks the best?

11. decode the menu, evaluating each item and the side dishes to see if you like each one?

12. pick an item but then tailor the item to your wishes (no mayonnaise, broccoli instead of fries, etc.)?

13. look up the menu online before you arrive at the restaurant, to see your options before you have a server waiting to take your order?

14. order according to your feelings in the moment, ordering healthy options or going wild depending on your mood?

15. order depending on your hunger level? If you're really hungry, anything goes!

Scoring

Your answers to the previous questions can help you assess where you fall on this spectrum:

Impulsive/ Spontaneous	Contemplative	Obsessive/ Indecisive

Increased Response Speed		*Decreased* Response Speed

2,3,12 13/4

▶

Questions 1, 4, 10, 14, 15: Impulsive/Spontaneous. You tend to make snap decisions, which keeps them interesting and varied. However, it's likely that your decisions are more emotion-driven—they depend on your mood at that moment. Your task is to take a mindful pause. This will help you get in touch with how you're feeling and give you time to weigh *all* the options.

Questions 3, 6, 11, 12, 13: Contemplative. You take your time to consider your options. This is great *if*, as you ponder the menu, you're able to integrate the options with your feelings (what you want) to arrive at an insight-driven decision. However, it's also possible to contemplate yourself right into an unhealthy choice because, well, you just want it. The good news is that you can learn to use your natural thoughtfulness to both think and feel your way to the healthiest option that will still please your palate.

Questions 2, 5, 7, 8, 9: Obsessive/Indecisive. Making decisions can be downright painful. You may overthink your options, push them onto your dining partner, or simply order what everyone around you is ordering. Relying on your gut instinct may help, too—asking yourself what you *feel* instead of what you *think*. Don't think too long, though; it may leave you paralyzed. There's no freedom in your dining partner making the decision for you!

Now that you know more about your decision-making style, the next time you make an eating decision, consider where you fall on the spectrum and slide yourself a little in either direction (unless you're in the middle). If you make impulsive decisions, make an effort to read every option, even if it's painful. If you obsess over your decisions, trust your gut a bit more.

Don't Fall into the Gap

Let's say one of your coworkers always brings doughnut holes to work on Fridays, and you tend to mindlessly pop them into your mouth. If I asked you to predict, right now, if you'll eat one (or more) this Friday, your response would depend, in part, on how you feel at this moment. If you're feeling good, you're likely to say no, you won't. But what if you don't feel as upbeat on Friday, when those doughnut holes are sitting on the break-room table?

Welcome to the *empathy gap,*[10] a term that describes your inability to imagine feeling any other way than the way you feel right now. If you've ever gone to the supermarket ravenous and bought way more food than you needed because you couldn't imagine *not* feeling ravenous, you've fallen into the empathy gap.

Perhaps you fall into the hot-to-cold empathy gap. If so, when you experience "hot" emotions (anger, stress, frustration), you're unable to consider that they will eventually pass. Similarly, if you experience a strong craving, you have to answer it *now,* without considering that it may fade.

If you fall into the cold-to-hot empathy gap, you tend to underestimate how much your hot feelings affect you in the moment. When you aren't experiencing a craving, you might find it hard to imagine how tightly your desire for chocolate or that fourth slice of pizza will grip you, how difficult it will be to manage a craving in the moment you experience it, and how significantly it will erode your ability to make an insight-driven decision. Because you underestimate how much hot feelings can hijack your decisions, it's difficult to plan to cope with them.

My clients discover this the hard way. For example, they may be casual about making a food plan, telling themselves, *I don't need a plan. I know what to eat.* At our next session, they tell me they caved in the day after our previous session. They are unable to imagine their calm, relaxed moods turning into frustration and anxiety, so they make emotion-driven decisions when stress or anger hits.

You can use your understanding of the empathy gap to help you more accurately perceive, predict, and prepare for how your emotions may sway your moment of decision. If you know you generally like a snack in the afternoon, acknowledge that desire, assume you will experience it, and pack a healthy snack so you won't need to hit the vending machine. You can prepare for feelings you know you'll experience, but you can't prevent them—anger toward a nasty supervisor, say, or your daily commute. Finally, when you're in the midst of an emotional food craving, you can remind yourself that it may pass and try to wait it out.

How do you manage to do all that? How, in fact, do you learn to make insight-driven decisions? During the moment of decision, you take a mindful pause. It can help you work through your first impulse: to react. Then you deploy the EAT method, which we'll discuss in chapter 3.

DEEP AWARENESS

A fundamental aspect of EI relates to your ability to perceive what you feel. To perceive your feelings is to know what you're feeling as you feel it. Mindfulness helps you develop this kind of awareness. If you've read any of my previous books on eating issues, body image, and weight, you know that mindfulness and awareness are the focus of my work with clients.

Mindfulness is being deeply aware of what you're thinking and feeling in the moment, in an open and accepting way. A centuries-old concept in the Buddhist tradition, mindfulness is both an experience and an attitude. It's tuning in to your mind, body, and thoughts like you might tune in to a station on an old-fashioned radio, twiddling the knob until you find that crisp, clear signal.

You may be thinking, *But I do know how I feel.* But mindfulness and emotional intelligence impart a different way of tuning in to your emotions, knowing not just what's in your head but in your body and mind as well.

Let's say you know you're feeling stress. This type of awareness helps you tune in to that stress on a deeper level—what thoughts it brings to mind, what feelings you experience as a result, and how those feelings "feel" in your body. As you experience the stress, you let it be, accept it without trying to control or judge it. Knowing your stress inside and out can be immensely helpful if stress tends to trigger a desire or urge to eat.

Sadly, we aren't too skilled at identifying and staying with our feelings. Our culture tells us to numb them, run away from them, escape from them, not tune in to them. We're not good at managing boredom either. Sitting still can be difficult. Mobile phones, computers, and social media have made it worse. Technology gives us little time to be alone and savor stillness or even the slightest pause. The moment of decision can feel uncomfortable.

Furthermore, because we live in a culture that values accomplishment and results, we've been trained to focus on the future rather than on the present. We don't know how we'll feel tomorrow or five years from now. We can only identify what we feel now. But those *now* feelings, be they positive or negative, shape the thoughts and behaviors that can affect our food choices in the present and the future. We act first and then ask questions later. But once we learn to respond, not react, we make wiser eating decisions.

A number of studies have found that mindful eating techniques help control cravings, reduce overeating, and promote weight loss without dieting. The emotional intelligence skills you'll learn in this book—a hybrid of emotional intelligence exercises and mindfulness techniques—can help you cope with everyday stresses and emotional triggers that drive you to eat. While simple to do, they are powerful alternatives to self-soothing with food.

Your Primary Keep-Calm Tool: The PAUSE Formula

In emotional intelligence theory, awareness is the key to improving the quality of your decision making, and a *mindful pause* (some of my clients call it "pressing PAUSE") can help you achieve it. Because it creates a gap between the impulse to eat and actually eating, this tool can help you

- become aware of the moment of decision,

- tune in to what you're feeling and your hunger level, and

- calm down, so that you can make a clearheaded decision.

Many people find it difficult to keep calm because they try to intervene at the cognitive level—that is, they direct themselves to "just calm down." It's more helpful to prevent your body from shifting into fight-or-flight mode, which raises your breathing and heart rate. Pressing PAUSE tricks your body into thinking you're calm by actively and intentionally slowing down your body, which gives you the opportunity to make an insight-driven choice.

You can use the PAUSE formula

- whenever you are about to eat,

- when you are struggling with a food-related decision (like whether to have a second helping),

- to assess your feelings in the moment you're experiencing them,

- to identify when you're stressed and you feel the urge to stress eat, and

- to respond calmly rather than react to your emotions.

Here's the PAUSE formula:

P: *Perceive.* Stop for a moment. Tune in. Identify this very moment as a moment of decision.

A: *Allow* at least ten seconds for that awareness to sink in.

U: *Understand* your feelings. First, sum up whatever you're feeling in two or three words (sad, mad, happy, frustrated). Next, ask yourself if your thoughts are being driven by insight or emotion. Finally, tune in to your body. Is it offering any clues about how you're feeling (clenched fists; slumped shoulders; rapid, shallow breathing)?

S: *Stay* in the moment. Do the focused breathing exercise on page 54. Notice any urge to push your emotions away (*I don't want to feel this!*). "Lean into" the feelings instead of away from them, asking yourself how you can use them to guide rather than push you.

E: *Entertain* your options. Give yourself at least two. They may address eating specifically (option A: eat another helping;

option B: skip it; option C: one more bite) or provide an alternative to eating that calms your body (a walk, a kickboxing class), your mind (a computer game, a crossword puzzle), or your spirit (prayer, meditation).

Pushing PAUSE can lead to a moment of insight. If you're a frazzled mother, perhaps your moment of insight is just that this one particular stressor, at this particular time of day, is here to stay. It won't change, at least for a long while. But it's predictable. You *know* it's your most vulnerable time of day. The solution to the problem is in the problem itself. Your "intervention" might be to invest in a slow cooker and a slow-cooker cookbook filled with healthy recipes, have a small but healthy snack before you get home, and throw a Frisbee or take a pre-dinner stroll with your kids as dinner bubbles away.

Beyond PAUSE: Four Core Keep-Calm Tools

Before we turn to the EAT method, let me introduce four other core tools to use in the moment of decision:

1. Tuning in to the now (a basic mindfulness meditation)

2. Calming words

3. Q-TIPP (focused breathing)

4. Peek behind the craving (understanding your triggers)

All these tools utilize the power of mindfulness and emotional intelligence. They'll help bring you into your mindful pause so you have the chance to make an insight-driven decision.

I'll refer back to these core tools (as well as pressing PAUSE) throughout the book, but they're so powerful that you can use them successfully today. Use one or all to regain a sense of calmness when you feel stressed, frustrated, or anxious. Whichever technique you choose, practice it for several minutes. Live in that gap between thought and action. Then, revisit your craving or desire to eat.

NUTRITION KNOWLEDGE COUNTS TOO

Your knowledge of nutrition can influence your eating decisions, too. That's why, to raise your Eat.Q., it's essential to know the basics of nutrition. The following table shows how Eat.Q. (high or low) intersects with nutrition knowledge (high or low). Read the profiles after the table to see which one sounds most like you. Remember, these are possible but not absolute outcomes.

	↓ Low nutrition knowledge	↑ High nutrition knowledge
↓ Low Eat.Q.	Weight gain, an unhealthy diet, emotional eating, mindless eating	Weight gain, an unhealthy diet, emotional eating, mindless eating
↑ High Eat.Q.	Weight gain, an unhealthy diet, mindless eating	Weight loss, weight management, mindful eating, a healthier diet

↓ **Low Nutrition Knowledge with a** ↓ **Low Eat.Q.**
Common consequences: weight gain, an unhealthy diet, emotional eating, mindless eating
You may fit this profile if . . .

your knowledge of nutrition is limited or needs to be updated. Or, because you are busy, you get the majority of your advice from supermarket tabloids or the diet guru of the moment. It's rare to get a solid education on nutrition in school unless you seek it out. The fact that you typically choose foods for comfort or convenience, rather than health, can also undermine your efforts. To sharpen your nutritional knowledge, try www.nutrition.org.uk, the website of the British Nutrition Foundation. For readers in Australia, visit www.eatforhealth.gov. au. You'll get current nutrition information from a credible source.

↑ **High Nutrition Knowledge with a** ↓ **Low Eat.Q.**

Common consequences: weight gain, an unhealthy diet, emotional eating, mindless eating

You may fit this profile if . . .

you know it's important to eat more plant foods (fruits, veggies, whole grains) than processed foods, and you differentiate between healthy carbohydrates and fats and those that promote weight gain and chronic disease. Lack of nutritional knowledge is not a problem. In fact, you might be an encyclopedia of nutritional facts. However, you may have difficulty managing strong emotions and are vulnerable to the what-the-hell effect and stress eating.

↓ **Low Nutrition Knowledge with a** ↑ **High Eat.Q.**

Common consequences: weight gain, an unhealthy diet, mindless eating

You may fit this profile if . . .

you generally don't overeat to soothe or comfort yourself but you believe you make healthy choices when you don't, often by accident. For example, the typical salad at a chain restaurant is large and loaded with high-calorie extras, such as bacon, cheese, croutons, and dried fruit. Not only is it loaded with artery-clogging saturated fat, it's extremely calorie-dense. You may be eating more than you think if you eat out frequently for business or pleasure. Tricky marketing techniques for foods like cereal, which claim health benefits but are packed with sugar, may trip you up as well. A solid education will help you separate nutritional fact from fiction.

The good news? Once you get the nutrition knowledge you need, you're already emotionally able to use them.

↑ **High Nutritional Knowledge with a** ↑ **High Eat.Q.**

Common consequences: weight loss, weight management, mindful eating, a healthier diet

You may fit this profile if . . .

> Actually, I don't expect you to fit this profile . . . yet. In many ways, it describes what you're aiming for—to blend your nutritional and emotional knowledge. The good news is that no matter which profile sounds like you, you can change it. While you may occasionally struggle with cravings or overeat, as almost everyone on the planet does, those slips will be fewer and far between once you raise your Eat.Q.— and everyone can stand to raise theirs a notch or two.

Keep-Calm Tool 1: Tuning In to the Now

Meditation is one action that can fill the space between a thought and an action—that all-important moment of decision. It focuses your thoughts and helps you stay in the moment. Both benefits are essential when you're trying to order from a menu, choose a snack, or ride out a craving. Practice the following technique whenever you're vulnerable to reacting rather than responding.

- When you feel overwhelmed and want to soothe your stress,

- when you're so furious you don't care what you put in your mouth, or

- when you feel listless and are tempted to eat for something to do:

    1. Find a comfortable, relaxing position. If you're at home, your favorite chair or bed is ideal. However, you can do this meditation anywhere, including your office chair or airplane seat.

    2. Intentionally place your thoughts in the present. Try not to think about the past or the future; stay focused on *this* moment. Say to yourself, *Be here*. Notice your attention zooming in to this moment.

    3. Shift your mind into one of non-judgment. Accept whatever thoughts come into your mind, positive or negative. Adopt a curious stance—as thoughts pop up, say (or think), "How interesting." Use your breath as an anchor to this moment. To tune out

distractions, focus on the movement of your chest as you breathe and on the sound of your breath.

4. Begin to watch your thoughts come and go. Allow them to be what they are. Take note of them without trying to change or alter them.

5. Let go of any thoughts that pop into your mind. Imagine them floating up to the surface of water, like a bubble, and popping or floating away on the surface. If you find your mind wandering to other things going on in your life, gently bring your focus back to your breathing.

6. When you feel ready, open your eyes. Prepare to shift your attention back to what you were doing.

With practice, mindfulness can be a mind-set instead of a meditation. I notice when I'm zoned in or zoned out; for me entering a mindful state is like shifting a lever. Before the shift, I'm listening to someone talking; after the shift, I'm listening to the sound of my breath leaving my nostrils. I become present in my body, and I quiet for a moment the chatter in my head. It's easy to get stuck in your head with worry. This moves you away from your head and into your body.

If you are unable to do mindful meditation to calm down, you can also try:

Keep-Calm Tool 2: Calming Words

Fill the gap between feeling (anger, frustration, sadness) and action (eating) by saying a silent prayer or a calming or motivational word, verse, or mantra. Here are a few examples:

- This too will pass.

- I will survive.

- I can make the best of it.

- It's not the end of the world.

- Keep calm and carry on.

Repeat for several minutes or until you feel calm.

Keep-Calm Tool 3: Q-TIPP

The practice of mindfulness raises your willingness to tolerate uncomfortable emotions. Q-TIPP, or focused breathing, is a simple and effective way to attain calm, even if you've never tried a mindfulness exercise.

In one study,[11] researchers at the University of California, Los Angeles, wanted to know whether focused breathing would help people feel calmer and more composed after they viewed a series of negative photos selected to elicit positive, negative, and neutral emotions. So, they broke sixty healthy young people into three groups. (All were screened by a depression and anxiety inventory, and none had undergone counseling in the previous two years.) The first group was taught focused breathing, the second was told to let their minds wander, and the third was told to worry about a multitude of things, including money, health, and achievement. Then each group was shown the photos.

In just fifteen minutes, compared to the worry and wandering-mind groups, the focused-breathing group reported fewer negative emotions and less emotional instability. In other words, this group's emotions remained on a fairly even keel. Also, the focused-breathing group was more willing to look for longer periods of time at the negative slides (such as a dirty toilet, snakes, a woman crying) than the unfocused attention groups. The volunteers in this group weren't scared of feeling bad; they were ready to face it head-on. Wouldn't it be nice to take some focused breaths and march toward whatever is bothering you instead of pushing it down with food?

FOCUSED BREATHING EXERCISE: Q-TIPP

An acronym for focused breathing, Q-TIPP, is particularly helpful when you're wrestling with yourself about whether or not to eat. The more you use this technique, the more quickly and easily you'll be able to make insight-driven decisions.

As you do this exercise, focus on the actual sensations of breath entering and leaving your body. Don't think about your breathing; just experience how it feels. If your awareness wanders, gently bring yourself back to the sensations of breathing.[12]

Q: *Quiet* your mind. Close your door, turn off your phone, walk away from your computer. Sit in a comfortable spot. Close your eyes. Empty your mind and let go of distracting thoughts. Focus on the present moment. If you can't stop what you're doing, that's okay. Just turn your attention to your breathing.

T: *Touch* base with your senses. Name what you hear, see, smell, taste, touch around you.

I: *Inhale* slowly and deeply through your nose. If you need imagery, imagine inhaling the fragrance of your favorite scented candle.

P: *Pucker* your lips and, *very slowly,* push out your breath.

P: *Pause* and hold for a moment.

Repeat this ten times. If you still feel stressed, repeat ten more times or until you're calm. *Then* make your decision.

Keep-Calm Tool 4: Peek Behind the Craving

If you're more of a thinker than a feeler, this tool may appeal to you. It taps into the analytical part of your brain so you can observe and understand what you're feeling, cool your impulses, and determine exactly why you want to eat.

Sometimes you want to eat because you're physically hungry. Other times, your "hunger" is a reflection of how you're feeling. The next time a craving blindsides you, buy some time by asking yourself these questions:

Where are you? In the kitchen? Your bedroom? Your office? Was the craving linked to your location? Can simply standing in your kitchen trigger cravings?

What are you doing? Working at the office? Doing laundry? Driving the kids to lessons? Hanging out watching TV or reading? Are there particular activities that activate your appetite?

How are you feeling at this moment? Name the predominant feeling you're having right now.

Who is with you? Or are you alone? Does the person you're with or your relationship tend to trigger cravings? Is he or she a helper or a hinderer (chapter 6)?

Why do you want to eat? Was your last meal or snack more than three hours ago? Are you looking for pleasure (chapter 5)? Are you overwhelmed by stress (chapter 7)? Are you feeling a particular way and want that feeling to stop?

Make it a habit to "peek behind the craving" every time one pops up. Before long, you'll ask yourself these questions automatically, which raises the odds that you'll respond rather than react.

No More Eenie Meanie Miney Moe

Ready to try an alternative to the snap decision? These tips can help. First, try the PAUSE formula and/or a keep-calm tool. Then, use the following tips to take you to the next step: choosing an option.

- *Limit your options.* Narrow your choices to just a few. When you have too many options, you run the risk of choice overload. In a classic study,[13] a Columbia University professor set up a booth of samples of jams at an outdoor market. Sometimes the professor displayed twenty-four jars of different jams, at other times just six jars. The larger assortment drew a bigger crowd, but more people bought the jam when they had only six choices (30 percent versus only 3 percent when they had the choice of twenty-four jams). Fewer options helped people decide to buy.

- *Make it routine.* Even in the midst of strong emotions, we tend to keep to our routines. For example, we brush our teeth regardless of how we feel because we brush our teeth every day. Similarly, having a routine healthy afternoon snack can remove the emotional struggle between hitting the vending machine and eating a snack that you packed at home. If you bring a snack every day, going to the vending machine will no longer be a habit.

- *Take options off your plate.* Knowing what you don't want to eat is as important as knowing what you do want. If you're having difficulty deciding, start with firmly ruling out what you don't want. For example, decide what restaurants you don't want to go to (no

Chinese food) versus what you might want (Italian, Thai). This can help rule out distracting variables (such as what your significant other wants you to eat or what you think you "should" eat) and clarify your decision-making process ("I don't want anything spicy").

- *Close your eyes.* Although you might feel silly, one study found that blocking out stimuli, even for a few seconds, helps you gain better access to an emotion.[14] (If you feel upset, you will know that you feel upset.) This technique also helps you visualize the problem. As I say time and again, to make insight-driven decisions, you must be clear on exactly what you're feeling.

- *Become okay with "good enough."* A chocolate-chip granola bar might not be an apple, but it's not a huge chunk of chocolate fudge either. There's something to be said for a pretty good decision sufficing, according to Dr. Barry Schwartz, a professor of psychology and author of *The Paradox of Choice*.[15] The good-enough stance takes the *I blew it anyway* feeling out of the decisions that lead to overeating.

- *Nudge your decisions gently.* Make the choice you want to make the most convenient option possible. In one canteen-line study,[16] making healthy options very convenient, in comparison to unhealthy options, significantly changed people's decisions. (Healthy food sales rose by 18 percent and less healthy food fell by 28 percent.) The choice was virtually made for them because people tend to opt for convenience. Thus, putting healthy food in very convenient places makes the decision a no-brainer.

The Last Bite

Maybe you've always known that your feelings lead you to food. Maybe that knowledge is just sinking in. Either way, take heart. Before long, you'll be able to identify the moment of decision, take a mindful pause, and respond rather than react to your feelings, which leads to healthier eating decisions. How does it feel to realize that you actually have a choice: to eat, or not? If that thought gives you hope, good! If it leaves you feeling apprehensive, that's okay too. Once you learn to use the tools in this chapter, which have helped so many of my clients move from reaction to mindful response, you'll find it much easier to make healthy choices.

In the next chapter, you'll learn how to use the EAT method to transform your relationship with food.

3

The EAT Method

Take Charge of Your Eating

If the only tool you have is a hammer, you
tend to see every problem as a nail.

—Abraham Harold Maslow

This quotation—the famed psychologist's metaphorical explanation of why people get so stuck when it comes to problem solving—fits the issue of overeating perfectly. So many people hammer at overeating with what they perceive as their only tool: dieting. This chapter invites you to try a new tool,

food for THOUGHT

- What methods have you used to lose weight and eat healthier? Which techniques were helpful, and which were not?
- Would you describe your feelings as intense and clear, or fuzzy and confusing?
- Are there particular emotions that cause you to shut down, making you unable to verbalize your feelings? For example, do you typically shut down when you're angry? Or do you react, yelling and stomping around?
- When you experience an intense emotion, how do you typically respond to it? Would you say your coping strategies are healthy, unhealthy, or both? Which strategies are healthy, and which are unhealthy?
- How might healthier eating change your life? How might it make you feel?

a three-step method I call *EAT—Embrace* your feelings, *Accept* them, and *Turn to* positive, non-food alternatives.

A combination of mindfulness and emotion-regulation skills adapted from the EI model, EAT helps you harness your emotional intelligence to alter your relationship with food and make healthy eating decisions. It can help you manage your eating, withstand cravings, and recover from slips or binges, even if you've struggled in the past. Here's your direction: increase your EI, and you increase your ability to stop emotional eating.

However, to make the best use of this new tool, you must be willing to see the "problem" of overeating in a new way. It's not a nail you can pound into submission with a hammer—that is, with dieting. It's a mind–body issue that restriction can't fix.

Often, before they try the EAT method, my clients have a myopic view of their struggles with food. They say things like:

"I'll never lose weight!"

"I'm such a failure at eating better."

"Why try? Diets work for a while but nothing ever changes. I always end up back in the same exact place."

Clearly, they're frustrated, tired of dieting, and have almost lost hope. Once they learn, practice, and fully embrace the EAT method, things begin to move in a better direction. They feel hope that they will finally enjoy food instead of constantly wrestling with it.

Yes, some of my clients see changes in their weight, which they are exceedingly happy about. But the change goes deeper than that. They become more confident around both other people and food; more sure of what they want, need, and value; more decisive; more "in charge" of their emotions; and more deeply aware of the connection between how they *feel* and what they *do*. Their tune changes to:

"I can do this."

"It's a process; it doesn't happen overnight."

"I need to step away from the scale and focus on building my confidence."

"It's amazing how when I stop letting my feelings be in charge, I generally don't overeat."

The EAT method is grounded in dozens of clinical studies published in top medical and nutrition journals, and these studies associate low EI with problematic eating (such as eating past fullness, turning to food when you're angry or bored, and overeating pleasurable foods on impulse). Conversely, research also suggests that learning skills to cope with feelings (and remember, you *can* learn them!) can help raise EI and reduce the tendency to eat emotionally.

EAT is a straightforward and systematic way to engage complex emotions. The next sections tackle it one step at a time.

The EAT Method

Step 1: Embrace Your Feelings
Mechanism of Change: Learning to notice,
identify, and feel your feelings

Typically, our minds are oriented toward the external world—what's in the news, our schedules, our challenges, or our plans. In this step, you learn to embrace your feelings by tuning in to them—to perceive, identify, and feel your feelings, whatever they may be. I often call feeling your feelings "welcoming them in," like saying hello to a guest coming in the door.

As you develop your ability to tune in, you'll get better at identifying and understanding the feelings that drive you to food; and the more you understand them, the better you'll manage them.

If you have a driver's license, you likely know what a blind spot is. When you're behind the wheel, the blind spot is the area outside your normal field of vision. You have to consciously turn your head to see it. Sometimes we humans have emotional blind spots, which we can't see unless we consciously look for them or someone points them out to us.

For example, one client, Erica, a teacher, got mad over little things. She was just wired that way. I knew it; her friends and family knew it; in fact, anyone within earshot knew it. Erica was clueless, although she *did* know that she heard a lot of "You're yelling again" from friends and family.

In our work together, Erica came to see that her constant irritability, and her loud declarations of that same irritability, constituted an emotional blind spot. Tuning in to the sound of her own voice (Was it normal? Raised? Was she yelling again?) helped her stay one step ahead of her irritability, which improved her relationships and reduced the number of times she picked up food when she felt upset or angry. Tuning in to her body, Erica found that it gave her clues that she was angry. For example, she trembled or got hot. Tuning in to her thoughts, her clue was a stream of swear words.

As you learn to embrace your emotions, your body can give you important information about what you're feeling, too. Trembling, rapid breathing, slumped shoulders, balled-up fists—your body language can be your first clue as to what's going on inside. (In chapter 9, we'll explore body language more fully.)

The E sections of the book and the E tools (chapter 9) may strike you as fairly easy. As the first building block of the EAT method, it's meant to be so. However, emotions are deceptively simple. They seem straightforward until you begin to peel back the layers and notice that some emotions occur on a conscious level while others hide at the level of your unconscious. Also, your

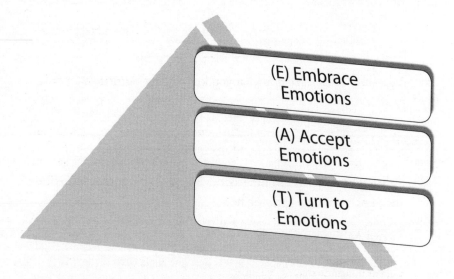

The EAT method rests on a foundation of becoming aware of, then fully embracing, your feelings. From that awareness, you learn to understand, accept, and manage them and ultimately turn to healthier alternatives.

body can give you conflicting information—maybe you're smiling at work when you're seething on the inside.

The Benefits of EAT: Weight Loss and Beyond

Will you lose weight if you learn the EAT method? If you're like many of my clients who stop mindless eating and emotionally driven eating, the answer is yes! Making discerning food choices, choosing more healthier options and fewer unhealthy options, and becoming aware of how your feelings influence your food choices all affect how much you eat. As a result, you lose weight, or your weight normalizes to a healthy range over time.

Studies on mindful eating have shown that being more mindful of your food choices and internal cues (hunger and fullness) leads to reductions in BMI[1] and caloric intake.[2] Plus, from an Internet survey of 17,000 dieters conducted by Roger Gould, M.D., of the University of California at Los Angeles, it's been estimated that 75 percent of overeating is caused by emotions. Therefore, just reducing emotional eating without making other changes has the potential to improve your health and weight.

The benefits of the EAT method extend beyond weight loss. Based on my experience with clients who have used the method, you can expect these additional benefits:

- Your body image will improve (when you eat better, you feel better about your body).

- You'll find it easier to put what you know about nutrition into practice.

- You'll actually enjoy eating again—food ceases to be your enemy and becomes one of the pleasures of life it was meant to be.

- When stress catches you off guard, you'll be better able to roll with the punches and go with the flow.

- As you learn to embrace your feelings, rather than fight or judge them, you'll enjoy closer, more loving relationships with your partner, children, and people in general.

- You'll be less self-critical. When you stop judging yourself, you'll enjoy life more and be less likely to turn to food to soothe yourself.

DOES SHIFTING YOUR MIND-SET MATTER?

A recent study conducted by experts in the fields of obesity and EI may be a game changer.[3] Its findings suggest that your state of mind may not only influence how physically satisfied you feel after a meal (researchers call this feeling satiety), but may actually change your body's response to the food.

The researchers focused on levels of ghrelin, the so-called hunger hormone in the gut, which stimulates appetite and feelings of hunger. Typically, ghrelin levels rise before meals and fall after you eat. Higher ghrelin levels in the system increase the likelihood of overeating.

In the study, the researchers gave all forty-six volunteers a 380-calorie milk shake. However, some volunteers were told that they were sipping a 620-calorie "indulgent" shake, while others were informed they'd received a 140-calorie "sensible" shake.

The participants who received what they thought was the indulgent shake experienced a dramatically steeper decline in ghrelin after they drank it. By comparison, the ghrelin response in those who thought they'd consumed the sensible shake didn't change. This flat response showed that despite receiving the same amount of calories as those who drank the indulgent shake, they were not as psychologically satisfied. The ghrelin response to perceived calorie counts matched what would be typical had the actual calorie counts been that high or low. In other words, although the participants drank exactly the same shake, those who thought it was an indulgent drink were more satisfied than those who thought it was sensible.

If you are trying to eat healthier, the finding that mind-set can affect satiety is important. In this study, the authors manipulated the description of the food. However, it happens all the time in the real world. Manufacturers label food items with terms like "low fat" and "healthy" or "decadent" and "sinful." These terms shape your expectations and consequently your satisfaction level. Now you know their trick! You don't have to let the label shape your expectations or appetite. Instead, think of a healthy meal or snack as a "treat"—it may help you enjoy it more and trick your body into feeling more satisfied.

The goal to lose weight can be fraught with desperation, frustration, and disappointment. Those negative feelings can interfere with the ability to use EI and develop a strong Eat.Q. For example, weighing yourself many times a week can interfere with your emotions. Step on the scale one day and you've lost weight—you feel elated. Step on it the next and you've gained a pound or two—instantly, that elation evaporates, and you feel terrible. As hard as it might be, please try to put specific weight-loss goals aside ("I must lose at least ten pounds"). Instead, trust that attempting the EAT method will bring you closer to all the benefits listed.

If you don't see shifts in your weight, please don't think you're doing something wrong. Sometimes medical issues, medications, or genetics play a role. For this reason, I encourage my clients to replace their weight-loss *goal* with a *commitment* to improve healthy eating. This change may not sound as appealing—at first. But it's a sure bet. Based on my clinical experience, if you eat healthier, you will definitely see changes—positive changes.

Putting Those Feelings into Words

An essential part of step 1 is learning the value of identifying your emotions with words. In fact, many of the E tools in chapter 9 are devoted to this skill.

Some of my more skeptical clients ask how this simple act can help them manage their eating and weight. I explain it this way: Imagine you're driving in your car, listening to the radio, when suddenly you lose the station. Loud, buzzing static fills the air. *Arrgghh!* Quickly, you switch off the radio to silence the painful racket.

That static is like a feeling, unidentified and chaotic. When the "racket" it causes inside you grows too loud to bear, you might silence it with food. Unfortunately, when the "painkiller" of food wears off, the static returns.

Now, imagine you're driving when the station plays a song you've never heard. Though unfamiliar, it speaks to you somehow. It draws you in. You turn up the volume and listen intently to the words.

Suddenly, you tear up—why, you don't know. Or a memory boils to the surface of your consciousness, something you haven't thought about for *years*. You're baffled: Where is this coming from? But it doesn't matter, because the lyrics perfectly capture your exact feeling. You hum the song, over and over. It becomes a part of you. Thereafter, when you're upset, it pops into your

WHEN THE WORDS WON'T COME

Words are the voice of the heart. —Confucius

We all struggle at times to verbalize our feelings. Emotions are complex and can be confusing, so they don't spring to our minds, or our tongues, with perfect clarity. However, people with alexithymia find it especially challenging to identify and express their feelings—skills central to EI and Eat.Q. I've worked with clients who have this condition, and in my experience, before their eating issues can be resolved, they must learn to find the words for how they're feeling. Fortunately, they *can* learn. And if you find it difficult to verbalize how you feel, you can learn too. Instead of stewing silently about a problem with your significant other, you'll be able to approach that person and say, "Honey, I'm upset. We need to talk."

There's good reason to learn. Healthy relationships with others, and with food, are built on the ability to identify what you feel and why, and the capacity to choose healthy ways to respond. An extreme difficulty verbalizing feelings, however, can cause significant problems in building healthy relationships and feeding yourself in a healthy way.

My clinical experience has shown me that the more people struggle with articulating their feelings, the more severe their issues with food tend to be.[4] People with high EI have a lower incidence of alexithymia, and vice versa. The following questions can help you decide whether you find it difficult to describe your feelings.

- Do you process what you're feeling while a situation or event is occurring, or hours or even days later?

- Do you shut down when you feel a strong emotion or prefer not to talk about it?

- When trying to describe how you feel, do you often choose the wrong words, perhaps saying that you feel "stressed" when you really mean "frustrated"?

- When you try to tell other people how you feel, do they not seem to understand what you're saying?

- Do you tend to have a lot of physical complaints (headaches, muscle tension, upset stomach)?

- Do you ever find yourself thinking, *Why bother trying to explain how I feel? No one will understand anyway?*

- Do your emotions tend to change from one minute to the next, making it confusing to know how you feel?

- Do you think more about how you feel than actually experiencing the feeling? For example, do you think about feeling sad, or do you experience sadness as heaviness in your heart or feeling torn up inside?

- Does your body send you confusing signals? For example, when your heart starts beating fast, you don't know if it means you're sick or upset.

- Do you sometimes feel an emotion that's different from what others think you "should" be feeling? Perhaps you feel mad when you lose something, when others think you should feel sad?

Because feelings can change rapidly based on mood and environment, a few yes answers is no big deal. If you answered yes to most of the questions, the tools in part 3 may help you improve your ability to put your feelings into words. If not, I recommend seeking a therapist who can help you develop the skills to talk about tough feelings. You might ask him or her to administer the Toronto Alexithymia Scale, which can give you an official determination of whether you have characteristics of this condition.

head. Instantly, you feel calm. Someone out there knows how you feel. You're not alone.

When you raise your EI, you find that "song"—the ability to put how you feel into the perfect words. The static is gone. Finding the right words calms you and helps you cope. The core keep-calm tools in chapter 2, plus the tools in part 3, will help you "tune in" and find those words.

Everyone has trouble tuning in now and again, but emotional eaters really struggle with it. When they can't tune in, their emotions tend to hijack their brains. Jackie was a client of mine who was just learning to use the EAT

HOW TUNED IN ARE YOU?

Being in tune with your body's internal cues (for example, noting that your heart flutters or your stomach knots up when you're nervous) is called *interceptive awareness,* and people who have it are more in tune with how they feel emotionally. Many studies measure interceptive awareness with what is known as a *heartbeat test.* For example, in a study published in *PLOS ONE,*[5] subjects in tune with their interceptive cues drank less water than those with low interceptive awareness—most likely, the researchers hypothesized, because they were more aware that they were full.

Want to see how tuned in to your body *you* are? Try the heartbeat test right now.

1. Set your phone or alarm to ring in one minute.

2. Close your eyes. Don't take your pulse or touch your body. Just try to tune in to your heartbeat.

3. Count the number of heartbeats you perceive during that time frame. At the end of a minute, record that number.

4. Set your timer again. This time, use your fingers to count. Write down this number.

This exercise isn't about getting the "right" number. It's about tuning in to your body and trying to perceive what's going on. If you can't perceive anything at first, keep trying. Each time you try to tune in, you're working on boosting your interceptive awareness.[6]

method, and her slip-ups with food had decreased significantly. However, one day she entered our session upset. She'd gone to dinner with her fiancé the night before, eaten half her entrée, and taken the other half home, a strategy we'd discussed and that she'd employed successfully several times. This time, however, still full from dinner, she'd polished off the leftovers.

"I don't even know why," she said. "I just blew it."

"What were you feeling just before you opened the refrigerator?" I asked.

"Well . . ." She sighed. "I was thinking about something Jim said at dinner, that maybe we should postpone the wedding until we're in better financial shape. To me, that sounded like he was trying to back out. At home, I kind of freaked out, and before I knew it, I was eating."

"So, how did you feel?" I asked.

"Um . . . anxious, I guess. I was really, really anxious."

I watched her face get that "look"—the look my clients get when they connect the dots.

When Jackie put her feelings into words, she understood that you don't just blow it. She ate because, in the moment of decision, she reacted rather than responded to an emotion: fear. Had she embraced that feeling— welcomed it in—she may have found it easier to press PAUSE and respond, rather than react.

Step 2: Accept Your Feelings

Mechanism of Change: Learning to use
emotions to help you think rationally and make
insight-driven decisions—choices based on a
combination of feeling and rational thought

Feelings are like a faucet. When turned on full blast, they can scorch or overpower you. Their flow is too forceful. When turned off, you don't get the water you need. Acceptance helps you adjust the faucet and manage the flow of your feelings. The first part of acceptance is to allow feelings in. Once you open to them fully and see what is there, you can put them to good use.

In this step of the method, you learn to accept your emotions so you can use them productively. And you do need to use them, because feelings are an indispensable part of making solid decisions. Your emotions can direct your attention to situations that demand immediate action. When you ignore, rationalize, or turn them off, you run the risk of not responding in an adaptive way.

Let's say you're on a holiday cruise, and you walk into the dining room and feel overwhelmed by the sheer volume and variety of food—too many choices, too much pressure to make the "right" eating decision. Unable to cope with the pressure aroused by the sight of the buffet, you shut it down with a rationalization—*I'm on holiday. Why not?*—and fill your plate to the brim more than once.

Unfortunately, emotional or stress eaters are experts at turning on the faucet full force, getting overwhelmed, and then shutting down the flow completely. One client, a paralegal named Mandy, was unusually honest

ACCEPTING WHAT YOU CAN'T CHANGE, CHANGES YOU

For after all, the best thing one can do
when it is raining is let it rain.
—Henry Wadsworth Longfellow

Acceptance—coming to terms with the reality of a situation without attempting to change it—is a central premise in many religious and spiritual beliefs, from Christianity to Buddhism. However, that doesn't mean it's easy. Struggling to accept the situation at hand has bedeviled humankind since the dawn of civilization; the Roman emperor Marcus Aurelius was quoted as saying, "Accept the things to which fate binds you, and love the people with whom fate brings you together, but do so with all your heart."

The notion of acceptance as part of treatment for overcoming alcoholism and other addictions has been around since the 1930s, most notably in Alcoholics Anonymous. The Serenity Prayer, written in the 1940s by theologian Reinhold Niebuhr and adapted for use by AA, is a key aspect of most twelve-step programs, including Overeaters Anonymous.

Only recently have we seen the notion of acceptance so clearly pop

about how well chocolate turned off her emotional faucet. "When my boss drops yet another pile of briefs on my desk, I feel like I just can't stand it," she said. "I get scared, pissed off, want to walk out the door and never come back. Chocolate is my medicine. It mellows me out and tunes out my stress better than any pill on the market. I hate that it works so well."

With time and practice, Mandy came to see that allowing, or accepting, your feelings is critical to directing your thoughts, which in turn will direct your behavior. Often acceptance comes from the ways your mind interprets and comprehends your feelings. As you learn to integrate your emotions with your thoughts, you'll make more insight-driven decisions. While accepting your feelings can be challenging at first, if you're will-

▶

up in treatments for eating. Psychologist Steven Hayes, the founder of acceptance and commitment therapy (ACT), champions acceptance as a key to change. It sounds paradoxical—you must accept where you are to be able to change—but evidence suggests that it works.

How might acceptance help manage eating? For one thing, it conserves a huge amount of emotional energy. Ever say to yourself, *Forget the chocolate on the top shelf—just don't think about it?* If so, you're engaging in *thought suppression*—trying to push down emotions and thoughts that are unmistakably there. When you try to forget about eating, research suggests that you actually think about it more, not less. Instead, acknowledging and accepting that you're having a craving actually leads to better success than trying to turn it off.

It's the same with feelings, which are messengers from your inner self. The more you struggle against them, the more powerful they become. The more you accept them, welcome them in, the less powerful they become—and, paradoxically, the more powerful you become. It will help you to know that acceptance isn't an event; it's a process. Part of the process is struggling with feelings and moving through them— exactly what the EAT method teaches you to do.

ing to tolerate a bit of discomfort, you'll learn to deal directly with all feelings—positive or negative—instead of using food to stuff them down or numb them out.

Although it wasn't easy, Mandy had to accept that, in her line of work, stress came with the territory. With acceptance came action. When her boss did his "folder drop," she was to sit quietly for at least one minute—acknowledging the stress, welcoming it in, using the core keep-calm tools and others in this book to sit with the anger, anxiety, and frustration that flooded her without lashing out at her boss or at herself with chocolate.

In time, she learned that feelings pass, and so do chocolate cravings. The more willing she was to accept that she didn't feel great, and that this was okay for a short time, the more she was able to withstand her cravings.

Step 3: Turn to Positive Ways to Manage Your Feelings

Mechanism of Change: Learning to manage
your feelings in positive, healthy ways

Getting over a painful experience is much like crossing monkey
bars. You have to let go at some point in order to move forward.

—C. S. Lewis

The T of the EAT method is very similar to the beautiful quote above: you let go of the past and reach for the next bar. While we all have healthy ways to manage difficult feelings—texting a friend, going for a brisk walk when you're angry, filling your down time and boredom with social media—the T tools offer new ways, based on the latest research.

At the moment, it may feel like eating is the only thing you can do to respond to an intense or overwhelming feeling. But this is not the case; you have options. Using these new tools is like coming in the back door instead of the front door. You've been trained to use the front door. It's direct, easy, and it works. The back door works too, but you may not know where it is. The T in the EAT method is that back door, giving you new alternatives to acting on your feelings.

The T tools focus on impulse control, distraction, imagery, and other creative ways to regulate your feelings. This *turning to* step teaches you to prevent or cope with cravings and use simple, clinically proven tips, techniques, and exercises to soothe yourself without food, develop food plans that you'll stick to, and make healthy decisions. The tools you'll learn are geared toward dealing with stress, which normally propels you toward the ice cream in the freezer.

Knowing what works for you is as important as knowing what doesn't. So, before you dive into this section, identify at least one healthy tool you currently use to cope with emotions that drive you to eat. It doesn't have to be grand and it may not work all the time, but we naturally gravitate toward certain kinds of tools. Do you lean toward those that involve using your body (cleaning the house, gardening, working out)? Or do you connect with others (calling or being with a friend)? Or do you employ cognitive strategies (making a to-do list to ease your stress and get things done)? Once you have that tool firmly planted in your mind, notice how it overlaps with the EAT method. Notice which emotions trigger you to reach for your go-to tool, what the feeling tells you about the need for the tool, and finally, what about it makes it successful for you.

For example, I have a client whose wife is a fantastic cook, so the refrigerator is always filled with pleasurable foods. When he works from home, his snacking increases tenfold. Working together, we devised a tool just for him: whenever he has the urge to boredom eat, he walks his dog. How many times he walks the dog on any given day tunes him in to other situations in which he has found himself going for the dog's leash—boredom was one feeling, but there were others, too, like frustration and being alone in the house (loneliness). Observing himself turning to positive alternatives, rather than to food, increased his confidence and helped him actually see how the EAT method works.

Identifying Your EAT Challenge(s): Andrea's Story

When I teach my clients the EAT method, my first task is to identify which part, or parts, they need to address. Some start with E—perhaps they've repressed or denied their feelings for so long they're emotionally numb. You need these feelings to help guide your actions and make positive decisions *consciously*. Others know how they feel and begin with A—accepting their emotions. Most of my clients need help with T—turning to positive alternatives to food or finding tools for coping with these emotions when faced with tempting treats or comfort foods.

At this point, you might ask yourself, *Where am I right now? Where could I use the most help?* Let me tell you about the experience of one of my clients, Andrea, who had the E and A down (boy, did she ever!) but needed help with T.

At our first meeting, Andrea knew exactly how she felt: furious! Three kids to care for, a demanding customer-service job, and an emotionally reclusive husband had brought her to the breaking point. Andy worked long hours, and when he arrived home, he zoned out. Andy had always been the strong, silent type. When they first married, Andy would "talk her down,"

IT BEGAN WITH A MARSHMALLOW: FINDING NEW TOOLS

Imagine this: I'm a researcher in a white coat and holding a clipboard. You're a subject in my study. I've put you in a room and seated you in a chair at a table. On the table is your all-time favorite food. (What is it? Pizza? Full-fat ice cream? French fries?)

As I head for the door, preparing to leave you in the room alone, I say over my shoulder, "By the way, don't eat that until I get back."

If you're like most people, this scenario elicits dread. But it happened to a group of four-year-olds in 1972 and involved . . . marshmallows.

As part of a now-famous Stanford University study, psychologist Walter Mischel gave four-year-olds one marshmallow and told them that if they could wait until he returned, they could have *two* marshmallows. You can still see black-and-white videos of this study on YouTube. While it's a hoot to watch little kids covering their eyes and talking themselves out of eating a single marshmallow, it's also slightly gut wrenching if you struggle with food.

Mischel's groundbreaking study gave researchers much insight into the delay of gratification and impulse control and the mind tools you can use to cope with the urge to overeat. Daniel Goleman's book *Emotional Intelligence* makes a convincing link between the ability to manage your impulses—the topic of Mischel's study—and life suc-

and for a while his emotional coolness helped Andrea manage her own feelings. Eventually, however, he got tired of that and tuned her out.

She, Andy, and food had gotten into a negative cycle. She'd feel overwhelmed by the kids, get irritated, and eat. Feeling bad about both the irritation and the eating, unable to cope, she'd turn to him for support. But unable to manage her stress and anger, her request for help came out as berating him for his lack of support. He'd tune her out. Feeling abandoned, helpless, and angry, she'd munch furiously at night, after the kids had gone to bed. Andrea would never turn this emotional eating around if she didn't

cess. To make it in life, along with a degree (perhaps) and hard work (always), you need the ability to cope and delay gratification.

Mischel's study is still relevant today, but in more ways than clueing us in to how to be an effective, successful leader. It gives us a framework for using EI to help us *eat* more successfully.

Let's return to the fantasy of you participating in my study. In some ways, you conduct this study every day of your life. You're alone in your kitchen with a bag of crisps. You're driving to work with a box of doughnuts on the passenger seat (it was your turn to buy them). You're at your desk promising yourself you can have the chocolate bar *after* you make that call or write that e-mail.

As it turns out, I'm not the one telling you, "Don't eat this now." Instead, it's *you* urging yourself to wait or not eat it at all. You're like one of those four-year-olds, only with a very—regrettably—grown-up dilemma: face to face with that treat, you must figure out how to control your impulse to eat, delay gratification, and manage all the feelings that arise from that struggle.

The T tools offer you solutions to that dilemma. Keep reading, and you'll be rewarded—not with a marshmallow, but with the ability to manage your emotions and impulses and make insight-driven decisions.

get a handle on the emotions that drove her to make unhealthy choices. Here is what her EAT process looked like:

E: Identifying and understanding her anger—what triggered it, how it felt in her body, and how it related to her eating. Being mindful of the early signs of anger helped Andrea deal productively before she tried to dampen her feelings with food.

A: Tolerating her anger. This is a tough assignment for anyone, including Andrea. We often want to push anger away or act out on it (by yelling, for example), which often makes things worse instead of better. By using a mindful pause and Q-TIPP to calm herself, Andrea learned to accept how she felt without guilt and manage it without a meltdown. Anger didn't have to always lead to overeating, as her mind tried to convince her time and again. In fact, the anger was a message. It was telling her that her relationship with her husband needed work.

T: Turning to new coping skills. Andrea needed new ways to deal more effectively with her anger and her husband. We brainstormed on the T part of the method, and she committed herself to *tuning in* and *turning to*.

The following diary page is an example of the type of journaling I ask my clients to do as they learn the EAT method.

ANDREA'S DIARY PAGE

E: *I'm angry again! I have really negative thoughts, and I'm pacing around the house.*

A: *This feeling will pass! Just let it be what it is. The more I tell myself not to feel that way, the more it doesn't work.*

T: *My gut reaction is to rummage around in the kitchen for a while or to yell at my husband, to get it all out. But, instead, I will cool down first so I can actually have a productive conversation. I'll do five minutes of Q-TIPP.*

At work, Andrea took the dish of sweets off her desk—no more de-stressing with chocolate. When boredom hit or an angry customer called, she played with one of the office toys she'd bought, practiced deep breathing, or repeated a soothing mantra she'd hung over her desk. These new skills followed her into the staff canteen. She used the EAT skills to choose healthier options instead of the foods that would please and comfort her palate at that moment.

At home, she learned to take strategic time-outs. She took a quick bath or went to her bedroom and shut the door for ten minutes. She stopped yelling at Andy and did something radical: she asked him for help, directly. When she asked him to supervise the kids at homework time, he did. When she asked him to fold the laundry, he did. But people aren't perfect; some nights he didn't. On those nights, some tasks fell by the wayside, and Andrea learned that this was okay.

Over a period of several months, as Andrea continued to *tune in* and *turn to,* her stress and dependence on food faded. She's become more accepting of herself, has a more easygoing approach to life, enjoys a more loving relationship with Andy and the kids, and shrugs off life's stresses more easily. Her life improved so dramatically, in fact, that Andrea considers the twenty pounds she lost a bonus.

Are You Ready for Change?

I must tell you that some of my clients are not quite ready to try or commit to the EAT method. It's not often, but it happens. The telltale sign is verbal resistance. They say things like "That won't work with me" or "I'll give this a try after my birthday." If they're exceedingly honest, they may even tell me "I'm not ready" or "I have too much going on right now." Or they give me that deer-in-the-headlights look. They may also have other issues they need to address first, such as a crisis or a more immediate problem, which we need to work on before we try the EAT method.

If this sounds like you, that's okay. Change isn't an event, it's a process, and there are several reasons you may not be ready to try this method quite yet. You may be alarmed about changing old habits, fearing that if you change one thing about your eating, your life might come tumbling down like a Jenga tower when you pull the wrong block. Perhaps you're unable to commit time to your own self-care—your relationship is troubled or you care for an aging parent or a house full of kids (even just one of these can be a handful). Or maybe your primary focus is on your physical or emotional safety. It can be tough to take care of yourself and your emotional needs if you feel you're in harm's way.

Are You Ready to EAT?

If you feel that you're just not ready, the following short exercise can help you identify the feeling that's blocking you from positive change. (If you're raring to go, you can skip this exercise.)

1. Sit in a quiet, comfortable chair or lie on your bed. Close your eyes. Imagine that you've started to make positive changes in your diet. Imagine yourself shopping for healthier foods, packing healthier snacks, turning down extra treats. Make these images as vivid and detailed as you can.

2. As your mind plays with these images, notice the feelings that emerge. Do you feel scared? Angry? Flat? Notice the strength of the images, too. Are they staying vivid or getting fuzzy? Are you unable to bring the images to mind at all? Do you see your spouse angry because his or her favorite snack isn't in the pantry? Do you feel afraid that it will be too hard or that you just can't do it? Even if the thoughts or images are negative, do you feel a tiny bit of hope or a feeling of determination?

3. As best you can, name the feeling that seems to be standing in your way. Fear? Resentment? A feeling of *it's not fair*? Discomfort or distraction due to an angry spouse? Hopelessness?

4. When you're ready, open your eyes and end the exercise.

Were you able to name a specific block? If so, your first step may be to devote time to removing it. If you feel fear, perhaps you can first line up supportive friends. If you're a caretaker, brainstorm ways to carve out time in your schedule. If your life is rocky at the moment, think of ways to get it in order so you can focus on your needs.

If you don't feel you're ready today, that's okay! Getting ready and just thinking about it is part of the process. Put it aside for a little while. Do some journaling about how you feel right now. Keep the book in a handy location so you can pull it out when you feel you're ready to take the next step. Or just flip through it now and commit to seeing how you feel in two weeks.

The Last Bite

I hope you're excited about the benefits of practicing the EAT method. There are so many, and they go far beyond simply losing weight. Practicing EAT makes you feel good, too, and when you feel good about yourself, you make healthier eating decisions. When you practice the EAT method, what you're really doing is accepting your feelings and making healthy choices regardless of how you feel. All the benefits of EAT flow out of this acceptance, and those benefits touch every aspect of your life, from your weight to your relationships.

In the next chapter, you'll learn about the first barrier to a strong Eat.Q.: dieting.

PART TWO

Barriers to Eat.Q.

Continuous effort—not strength or intelligence—
is the key to unlocking potential.

—Winston Churchill

My dictionary tells me that one definition of *barrier* is something that obstructs or impedes. My experience as a psychologist tells me that with enough self-compassion, determination, and courage (sometimes just enough!), you can overcome many of the emotional barriers that bar you from the life you desire and deserve. That's true even for emotional eaters, and even if those barriers were erected in childhood and have come to seem immovable.

In my experience, five common obstacles that emotional eaters face are dieting, pleasure seeking, social eating, stress, and trauma. These barriers can challenge even those who don't struggle with food or their weight. For emotional eaters, however, they can be especially troublesome.

That's because in varying ways each barrier affects the ability to perceive, understand, use, and manage feelings. Dieting distorts feelings around food and eating to the point that the feelings become secondary to the basic rules of dieting: restrict (food) and resist (desire). Pleasure seeking—in itself a normal, healthy drive—can become too strong, so that short-term desires (doughnut!) typically win out over long-term benefits (health, weight). Social eating is particularly difficult without healthy boundaries; if your boundaries are not as strong as they could be, you're vulnerable to food pushers, social anxiety, and a desire to fit in. When you're stressed, you typically react rather than respond to your emotions, and your ability to make sound decisions—about food or anything else—takes a huge hit. And trauma skews your emotions to such a degree that you can't understand or trust them—they're either too intense, too blocked, or simply too confusing.

Since you're reading this book, it's likely that you struggle with one or more of the barriers in this section. Can you acknowledge that? More important, can you accept it? That acceptance is crucial. If you can't acknowledge that a barrier exists, you can't very well knock it down! Read that opening quote again. How does it feel to read it? Does it apply to you? In a strange way, what feels like your weakest moment can be the moment of your greatest strength, if you work through it. So, take a deep breath. We'll tackle each barrier, chapter by chapter, so that you understand how your emotions play a role in each and how the EAT method can begin to remove them. Before long, you'll amass the skills you need to overcome the barriers and begin making decisions fueled by insight rather than emotion.

4

Dieting

The second day of a diet is always easier than the
first. By the second day, you're off it.

—Jackie Gleason

Do you recall hearing about the children's book *Maggie Goes on a Diet*? I do.
It was the talk of the office. With a reading level initially pegged to kids aged
four to eight, the book tells the story of a fourteen-year-old who is teased
about her weight. In response, she goes on a diet (albeit a healthy one) and
begins to exercise. She sheds the weight and becomes a football star, and her
popularity and self-esteem soar.[1]

---

food for THOUGHT

- What types of diets have you tried, and where did you find them? (In a weight-loss
  book or a magazine? Perhaps you got them from your doctor?)
- At what age did you begin to diet, and for what reason? Bullying? Competition?
  Following a parent's lead? Health reasons? How did you feel when you began that
  first diet? Sad? Anxious? Angry?
- Were your diets generally successful or not successful? How did *success* and
  setbacks feel to you?
- How does dieting affect the way you think? When you're overly hungry, do you
  start to obsess about food? Does doing so clear your mind?
- When you're on a diet, how do you feel physically? Emotionally?

It was a happy ending—for Maggie, at least—but for adults the book tapped into deeply negative feelings about dieting. The public outcry was so loud it made the news in the US.[2]

Although I believe the author's intentions were good and that he sincerely wanted to help kids cope with weight issues, I think something deeper was playing out. At a gut level, real people understand the cold reality of dieting: in the long run, it doesn't work.

At this point, we need to differentiate between improving the quality of your diet and/or having a healthy food plan—a good thing, given the rise in weight-related health problems—and *dieting*. The dieting I'm referring to is based on a very restrictive model (such as cutting out a food group or feeling deprived). Statistics on dieting show that the success of dieting is fleeting. A third to a half of everyone who loses weight regains it within a year.[3]

In my view, Maggie has an alternative to dieting. She can use EI skills—flexibility, impulse control, self-awareness (of her hunger and the emotions that urge her to eat), and self-regulation (finding healthy ways to cope with feelings). I think a fourteen-year-old can learn to do this; I think you can, too! In this way, you're set free from dieting and empowered to make a conscious choice about whether or not to eat.

As you read this chapter (and this book), I encourage you to examine your feelings about dieting, to really search your soul. What feelings does dieting elicit in you? How many times have you been on a diet billed as "the last diet you'll ever need"? Are you willing to consider an alternative approach to weight loss or weight management that involves not tracking calories or grams but your moods and feelings?

Living in *diet mode,* as I call it, can be frustrating. Often, the more you restrict your diet, the more you obsess about food. With every diet, you lose more trust in your ability to use internal hunger cues to tell you when to stop or start eating, and your thinking about your eating and weight becomes more rigid rather than more flexible. This rigid, all-or-nothing thinking can be dangerous.

As we've learned, the ability to be flexible is critical to EI and Eat.Q. My goal is to help you exit diet mode—the emotion-driven state of mind that persuades you that merely restricting your food intake will result in permanent weight loss—and enter Eat.Q. mode. There's a world of difference. Diet mode is "you feel it, you eat it," while Eat.Q. mode is "you feel it, you use it."

From Black-and-White Thinking to Shades of Grey

Many of my clients started out like Maggie: they went on their first diet, and it was good. Then, at some point, the diet failed them. They tried another . . . and another . . . and another, with diminishing success. Before they knew it, their feelings around food and eating had become secondary to the rules of dieting: the rules of restriction and resistance. They were trapped in diet mode.

In diet mode, you generally make decisions about what to eat based on the rules of any given diet (No sugar! No dairy! No wheat!). There are few allowances made for how you feel. Based on my experience working with clients, dieting can lead to psychological struggles around food—being afraid to eat; worrying excessively about what you did, did not, or want to eat; feeling guilty; counting calories; eating emotionally. It can also lead to disordered eating, which includes meal skipping and binge eating.

But you can use your emotional intelligence to help break out of diet mode. In Eat.Q. mode, you begin to see shades of grey: healthy eating isn't based on rigid rules but on a combination of flexibility and pleasure. By teaming emotion with logic, *you* decide how much and what to eat and respond to your cravings in a mindful way. You also learn to manage impulses and work through difficult feelings, so they don't drive your decisions. In other words, there's a difference between restricting and being mindful.

To further illustrate the difference between dieting and Eat.Q., imagine dining at a restaurant that features a dessert bar. You love desserts. They're your Achilles' heel.

In diet mode: *That dessert bar is calling my name. Oooh . . . they have raspberry cheesecake! No, no, no—I'm on a diet, and fat enough as it is. But it looks so good . . . but I can't. Oh, who am I kidding? I'll always be fat. The hell with it. Might as well eat it.* (This is an emotion-driven decision.)

This scenario is not likely to end well. As you'll see in a moment, dieters who try to suppress their thoughts about food frequently give up and give in. But there's another way.

In Eat.Q. mode: *That dessert bar is calling my name. Oooh . . . they have raspberry cheesecake! Sure, I want it. In fact, I want every dessert on the table. But I don't let my desire for sweets rule me. I'll eat my salad and dinner first and then see how I feel.* (This is an insight-driven decision.)

In diet mode, your impulse is to either resist your hunger or go overboard. In Eat.Q. mode, you counter that impulse by learning to become aware of how you feel in the moment. This awareness allows you to make a decision. Because you're not using emotional energy to resist the dessert table, it becomes easier to make a decision on how much to eat. True, it's not easy to determine how to eat "just a little" of something you love to eat. However, when you become more flexible in your thinking, it is possible to find a happy medium between eating too much cheesecake and none at all.

Let's examine the differences between diet mode and Eat.Q. mode more closely.

THE EAT METHOD MODEL OF DIETING

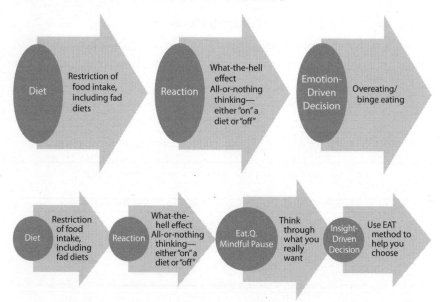

In diet mode, you restrict food. Feeling overly deprived may lead you to all-or-nothing thinking and giving up. In Eat.Q. mode, rather than act on the complex emotions that dieting can trigger, you use a mindful pause to help you avoid extreme thoughts and make solid decisions.

QUIZ: HOW DEEP IN DIET MODE ARE YOU?

Do you eagerly embrace every new weight-loss plan that comes out, reject dieting completely, or fall somewhere in between? Even if you don't diet often, you may still approach food and eating in diet mode (experiencing anxiety when you have cravings, overeating at a party, bingeing out of boredom or stress). The following short quiz can help you get a handle on your feelings about dieting in general.

1. How often do you think about dieting?

    a. It's always on my mind.

    b. Every now and then I ponder it, or at least eating healthier.

    c. It rarely crosses my mind.

2. When you spy a tempting treat, the first thing to pop into your mind is . . .

    a. I can't have it; it's not on my diet.

    b. I wonder how many calories (how much fat, how many carbs) it has?

    c. Diet or no, there's no way I'm passing *that* up!

3. In line at the supermarket, you see a tabloid headline: "Lose Ten Pounds in Ten Days!" You . . .

    a. toss the magazine on the conveyor belt. You're in!

    b. pick it up and flip to the article quickly, on the off chance it contains something new, and then put it back.

    c. ignore it and keep placing your items on the conveyor belt.

4. When you see a weight-loss gadget on TV, you think . . .

    a. I really need that (even if you don't buy it).

    b. I have one just like it, and it didn't work (or I never used it).

    c. What a gimmick.

5. Do you read stories about celebrity weight losses and gains?

    a. Always. I love to see celebrities gain weight—and lose it, too.

    b. I flip through the stories but doubt that the celebrities are losing weight in a healthy way.

    c. Never. The stories hold no interest for me.

SCORING

Give yourself zero points for each (a) answer, one point for each (b) answer, and two points for each (c) answer. Regardless of where you fall in the point spectrum, it's time to open up your mind to something new.

0–3 points: Hard-Core Diet Mode. Many of my clients fit into this category. Don't feel bad. You're about to learn a new way of thinking about dieting, which delivers solid, long-term results. Be prepared, though: if you've been dieting for most of your life, it may take time to let go of rigid food and diet rules. Once you learn the EAT method and use the tools in part 3, you'll be operating in Eat.Q. mode sooner than you think.

4–7 points: Diet Observer. Perhaps a veteran of the diet wars, you've learned that many popular or fad diets out there are hype, are unrealistic, or deliver only short-term results. Furthermore, you take new dieting information with a grain of salt, which is wise. Even so, old diet rules that you follow consciously or unconsciously may be holding you back. The EAT method will help root them out, so you can get the long-term results you're holding out for.

8–10 points: Diet Skeptic. It's likely you've been disappointed by diets too many times to risk getting burned again. You have no time or patience for gimmicks; it's the science behind weight loss that you want. You may even be skeptical of the EAT method. If so, read on. Voluminous amounts of research support the benefits of conquering emotional eating.

Difference 1: In diet mode, you track numbers.
In Eat.Q. mode, you track emotions and hunger.

In essence, dieting is a numbers game. This much lean red meat, that much grapefruit, this much ice cream, that much grilled chicken breast. Whether you track calories, fat grams, carbohydrate grams, points, or units of measurement (a tablespoon), a diet is all about the numbers. Even when a diet promises that you don't have to count numbers, it's because they've already been counted for you.

True, numbers matter. The twenty-nine grams of fat in a Big Mac is far too much if your goal is to manage your weight and protect your health.[4] But frankly, you have to manage the emotion-driven decision to eat it (the *I want it!*) before you can consider the numbers objectively.

Each time you decide what to eat, you choose based on your feelings—what looks good, what appeals to your eyes or your mood. If this were *not* the case—if you chose what to eat based on your knowledge of what you "should" eat—restaurant menus would be lists of nutrition facts rather than vivid descriptions using words like "sizzling," "succulent," and "buttery."

To illustrate the powerful emotions food raises in us, I offer exhibit A: a rather disturbing study conducted in the mid-1980s in which food researcher Paul Rozin, famous for examining the relationship between disgust and food, offered volunteers fudge in the shape of dog poo. *Ewww.* More than 40 percent declined it. They didn't think to themselves, *Hey, it's fudge.* Their emotion—disgust—clearly overrode their logic.[5]

Another excellent example of emotions rather than numbers determining our eating decisions was first observed by esteemed researchers Janet Polivy and C. Peter Herman. Their "what-the-hell" effect describes a cycle of behavior common to dieters—restrained eating (dieting) followed by overeating, guilt, and more overeating.

Polivy and Herman knew from previous studies that dieters use a tremendous amount of cognitive energy (aka, "willpower") to restrain themselves from eating the foods they want. So, in a seminal study on the phenomenon of *counter-regulation*—when people on diets are more likely to overeat than people who aren't—they compared how much ice cream dieters and nondieters ate after being fed either a small or a large milk shake. (A third control group received no milk shake at all.)[6]

They found that the dieters actually ate *more* ice cream after they drank the large milk shake than after drinking the small one. Why? Because even after the small treat, the dieters thought, *What the hell. I blew my diet anyway, so I might as well eat what I want.*

Studies have found that the effect crops up when dieters observe someone else overeating and even when they think—but don't know for sure—that they consumed a few extra calories. One study found that just *smelling* food led to the effect.[7]

What about you? Does the what-the-hell effect come out in you if, while on a diet, you give in and have a small scoop of ice cream or, instead of your grilled chicken breast, a slice of pizza? Chances are the answer is yes. If you've gotten to the point of saying, "The hell with it," you're undoubtedly dealing with a lot of emotion—shame, guilt, regret, anger, frustration, hopelessness. This is how easy it is for feelings to throw us off course.

Short-circuiting the what-the-hell effect is part of what the EAT method is all about. As you work on your Eat.Q., you're better equipped to deal with emotional eating.

MY MOTHER RAISED HER EAT.Q. . . . IN 1980

Writing this chapter, an image flickered in my memory: my mother's bookshelf in my parent's bedroom. Every bestselling diet book published in a twenty-year span shared space with the Bible and Danielle Steele, some of them dog-eared; others, as far as I can recall, she never opened. Spurred by this image, I visited my mother, who lives an hour away, to look at family photos and talk dieting.

As we sifted through photos at the kitchen table, we found one of her at a relative's wedding in New York City taken in the early 1980s, when I was in my teens. She shimmered in a little black number, one-shouldered, shot through with silver sparkles. "The ice-skater dress," as we'd called it, was extremely flattering—my mother was gorgeous and still is—and, for her, very daring.

She picked up the photo and laughed. "I looked great!," she said.

I heard her surprise and smiled. My clients have taught me that how you looked doesn't always match how you *thought* you looked, particularly when you're looking at an old photo.

A petite woman, my mother fluctuated between two sizes, and sometimes wanted to be in the smaller of the two. Although of Italian descent, she was your typical American woman: occasionally on a diet. As far as diets go, she played the field, so to speak, until she fell hard for the Scarsdale diet, published in 1978 by the late cardiologist Herman Tarnower.[8]

"That one wasn't on your shelf," I said. "You kept it in the kitchen, right next to the can opener."

"What better place for it?"

To this day, thirty-plus years later, she remembers that Monday lunches were a variety of cheese slices. (The current Scarsdale diet has been modified from the original version.) Her "perfect" diet did have one flaw, she said: You had to eat exactly what it said, when it said. Absolutely no deviations were permitted, save the default lunch of cottage cheese and fruit, which you could "enjoy" every day.

"Dr. Tarnower tried to help so many people," my mother said. "I remember the night I heard the news. I was watching TV in the kitchen, waiting for your father to come home from work." My father, a veterinarian, worked late shifts. "I had the news on, and they said Dr. Tarnower had been shot. I started to cry."

As she continued with her story, she said something electrifying, at least to me. As she sat at the kitchen table, shocked by the gruesome news, she'd been nibbling puffed-wheat cereal. It was not allowed on the Scarsdale plan, but she *always* ate it when she dieted. (So, yes, she "cheated," and with a food she didn't even enjoy. For her, as for most dieters, to diet is to cheat.)

With Dr. Tarnower's tragedy fresh in her mind, she felt guilty about eating a food forbidden on his plan. "That got me wondering: why was I eating it? And it came to me in a flash: because I was bored. I never overate during the day—only at night, sitting in the kitchen with nothing to do, waiting for your father. All those years of dieting, and that one simple thing never occurred to me."

Not long after that, she moved all her diet books—including the Scarsdale diet—to the basement. ("Oh, they're gone. I threw them out years ago," she said.) She still waited at the table for my dad to walk through the front door. But instead of watching TV, she read the latest thriller or pop psychology book.

My mother still reads at the kitchen table. What she doesn't do is nibble. Oh, magazine weight-loss success stories still pique her interest. But she learned long ago that she'll always be a "boredom eater" and she needs to stay aware and ahead of that emotion.

What better example of the difference between external change (diet mode) and internal change (Eat.Q. mode). When my mother pursued her moment of insight to find out where it led, she made a lasting change.

Difference 2: In diet mode, you follow rules.
In Eat.Q. mode, you listen to your feelings.

A friend recently lost a lot of weight on what she calls "a crazy, stupid liquid diet." In her eyes, it was successful: she lost over thirty-five pounds. But when we discussed this, she said something that made me prick up my ears.

By chance, she'd begun her diet just as her husband had been diagnosed with advanced skin cancer. As you can imagine, the bottom dropped out—her life felt completely out of control. Her appetite plummeted from worry. And although I can't prove it, I wonder if sipping shakes multiple times a day might have had a soothing, ritualistic quality in the midst of all that chaos.

Well, the good news is that her husband recovered. The bad news? My friend regained all the weight she'd lost, plus ten pounds.

When you're in diet mode, restricting calories or food groups or sipping shakes often gives you quick results, if you can tough it out. But even if you can, what happens when you're presented with an unexpected change to your schedule? What if you can't get your low-fat yogurt or mix your shake?

Yes, you can plan for contingencies (and all diet books tell you to plan), but it's been my experience that people tend to freeze when presented with situations that upend their diets or put them in proximity to "forbidden" foods. I remember one of my clients following the Atkins diet and doing quite well . . . until she volunteered at a pizza fund-raiser.

When you operate in Eat.Q. mode, you don't manage food; you manage your emotions, which in turn manages your cravings. As you raise your EI, you become more flexible in your thinking. You can take a pause and assess how you feel. You turn to positive alternatives.

For example, had my client been operating in Eat.Q. mode, she would have acknowledged that she would likely eat too much pizza and sent her husband instead (who no doubt would have enjoyed the pizza). Or she could have chosen to volunteer behind the scenes rather than on the "front line." But because she couldn't face that she was dying for pizza, she couldn't manage her cravings.

If you still don't buy that managing your emotions is the key to making peace with food, here's another story: Among my clients who are emotional eaters, several have had gastric bypass surgery. All of them lost weight—at first—but not all of them were able to overcome their emotional eating. Sadly, for them, the weight came right back on. Sometimes surgery can't fix the powerful impact of emotions on food choice.

This doesn't have to be you. When you live in Eat.Q. mode, you don't make drastic changes to your diet. You change the way you relate to food. One of the biggest changes is that you learn to adapt to a variety of situations. So, whether you travel to another country, go on a cruise, or simply can't get your hands on a low-fat yogurt or a meal-replacement shake, you'll do the next best thing: eat a sensible, healthy meal and go on with your life.

Difference 3: In diet mode, you fight your cravings.
In Eat.Q., you accept them.

Ever notice that as soon as you start your diet of the moment, you have cravings for foods that it forbids? On a low-carb diet, you crave pizza, bread, and potatoes. On a low-fat diet, you dream of succulent, fat-marbled ribs. And on almost any diet, your very soul cries out for ice cream, chocolate, or french fries.

What is that about? Simple: you're living the truth of the statement "What we resist persists." The more you resist something, the more your desire for it grows.

Time and again, studies show a strong link between food restriction (or dieting) and cravings. In a recent study in the journal *Appetite,* 129 women in three groups—those who were dieting to lose weight, those who were "watching" their weight, and non-dieters—recorded their cravings each day in a food diary and performed a daily mood assessment over a week's time. Compared with non-dieters, dieters experienced stronger cravings that were more difficult to resist. Not surprisingly, they craved foods that they "couldn't" have.[9]

Numerous studies have found that "control" strategies aimed at reducing unwanted thoughts or feelings tend to actually increase how often these thoughts or feelings occur and how long they last. However, an offshoot of such strategies, called acceptance and commitment therapy (ACT), takes a different tack. Instead of replacing negative thoughts, as you do in cognitive behavior therapy (CBT, a treatment that helps people understand how their thoughts and feelings influence their behavior), you accept them—make friends of them, if you will—which reduces their impact.[10] This approach has been shown to be just as, if not more, effective. Less of your emotional energy is used to struggle against yourself. (You will learn acceptance tools related to the ACT theory in part 3.)[11]

Resisting thoughts—such as thoughts about eating chocolate—can lead you to engage in the very behavior you wish to avoid. Researchers at Drexel University gave ninety-eight study participants a questionnaire to determine how susceptible they were to food urges, then gave them see-through boxes of chocolates to keep with them, night and day, for the next forty-eight hours. Those who fought the temptation to eat the chocolate used an acceptance-based strategy the researchers had taught them: admit and accept the craving, then choose not to act on it.[12]

When you make friends with those thoughts and let them come and go as they will, they lose much of their power. So, feel free to think about chocolate. Just use self-talk to dial down the cravings from "hot" to "cool" instead of trying to turn them off, and lose critical thoughts, such as *These cravings are killing me. I have no willpower. I'm such a loser.* These suggestions sound counterintuitive, I know. But cravings are like quicksand. The more you struggle, the more you sink.

Difference 4: In diet mode, you often feel drained and stressed.
In Eat.Q. mode, you are more likely to feel energized and calmer.

My client Sandra has a sign on her desk. It says, DOG NO PROBLEM. BEWARE OF DIETER. Like most jokes, it contains a grain of truth: when she's on a strict diet, this normally warm, funny, pleasant woman morphs into an absolute witch (her exact words), and a foggy-brained one at that. The sign works wonderfully (and I'm sure her colleagues appreciate the warning).

Perhaps you can relate. No one goes on a strict diet and becomes jollier. The fact of the matter is that dieting is hard on your moods, because it works against hunger instead of with it. In part, the crankiness is due to low blood sugar—it drops when you restrict your diet.[13] But the irritability may be more related to the *process* of dieting, and the issue is self-control.[14]

Like freshwater, lumber, and gold, self-control is a limited resource. You tap it many times a day as you deal with difficult people, maintain calm in stressful situations, and make healthy food choices. When you exhaust that daily supply of self-control, it's harder to manage feelings like anger and aggressiveness according to Dr. Roy F. Baumeister, a psychologist known for his research on self-control and coauthor of the book *Willpower.* Each time you exert self-control, no matter what the task (skipping a treat you really want or being unable to use the bathroom right away), you deplete your emotional resources. This is why at the end of the day, after stifling the urge to yell at a shop assistant and turning down a doughnut at a breakfast meeting, your resources are sapped and it's much harder to say no to cravings.

Dieting also makes it difficult to access emotional intelligence. When a client steps into my office and tells me he or she just started a strict diet, I expect we're in for an initial tumultuous session, filled with crankiness or downright anger. (Once that person gets used to these plans, irritability seems to fade.) Although sometimes that unfiltered

SARAH'S STORY

Sarah made an appointment with me not long after her fortieth birthday and spent much of her first session talking about the diets she'd tried. But under my gentle questioning, she began to touch on her feelings. For her birthday, her husband had thrown her a surprise party. When she blundered into the dark hall, startled by the triumphant shout of *"Surprise!"* a wave of gratitude washed over her—all the people who loved her were there, demonstrating their love in the most public way. That was the best part.

The worst part followed right on its heels. Among the balloons, flowers, presents, and bottles of champagne stood a three-tiered, elaborately decorated cake. She closed her eyes and made her wish. As she blew out the candles, her throat tightened and a tear slid down her cheek.

"My wish was, 'Please let this diet work so I lose weight this year,'" she told me. "Then I realized something: I've made this same wish for the last twenty years. That crushed me. But incredibly, my next thought was *And I'll blow my diet again tonight, when I have a piece of this cake.* Here I was at this amazing party, thrown *for me,* and I was fixated on my diet."

"Maybe dieting isn't the best path for you," I ventured.

She stared at me. "Isn't that how you lose weight?" she asked. "I came here to lose weight, right?"

"Has dieting helped you lose weight in the past?" I asked.

"Sometimes," she replied. "I've lost over twenty-five pounds on some diets. But then again, there have been times I've dieted and actually gained weight."

"Why?" I asked, although I had a pretty good guess.

"When I cheat, I feel incredibly guilty and beat myself up," she said. "The slightest slip and I'm like, *Well, I've blown it; might as well have some ice cream.*"

"What would it be like to just stop dieting?" I asked.

Sarah paused, considering. "Strange," she said, finally. "I've never *not* been on a diet. When I start the next one, I actually feel happy, like I'm doing what I should be doing."

For many sessions, we just focused on identifying her feelings about dieting: her anger about diet after diet failing her; under the anger, grief; feeling weak, on edge, even enraged. It took some time, but Sarah began to understand that she'd spent twenty years trying to win at what was, for her, a losing venture. It was a great day when Sarah confessed, "When I'm on a diet, I hate everyone around me. I have to starve myself to lose a pound, but the skinny girl at work can eat cheeseburgers every day. I hate her for that."

A month or so later, Sarah skipped her session. I don't call clients if they are doing well; I wait to see if they pop up again. Weeks later, she called—not for an appointment but to tell me something.

Her sister had come into town last week, she told me. She'd been dieting, as usual, but stopped when her sister arrived. "I decided to try Eat.Q. mode," she said. "I had no choice—my sister loves to eat like I do, and there's no dieting when she's in town. So, I did what we talked about. Every time I looked at a menu, I asked myself, *How do I feel? Starving? Satisfied? Do I want this appetizer because I love it or because I had a rotten day at work?* I pressed PAUSE, then ordered based on how I felt. Most of the time, I actually wanted to make the smart choice."

She'd lost two pounds, she said, even though they'd eaten out almost every night.

Although Sarah never returned to counseling, apparently everything we'd talked about made sense when she was ready to risk a new approach to eating. It was the first time she stepped out of diet mode and into Eat.Q. mode. I'm hopeful it wasn't the last.

negativity can lead to a breakthrough or an epiphany, it can be difficult to determine whether a tumultuous mood is due to what's going on in the person's life or the feelings of deprivation and irritability brought on by dieting.

Many of us would generally agree that it's important to follow a healthy

DIETING-INDUCED DIMNESS

You forget where you put your keys. You trip over your words. It's tough to form a coherent thought. Quite simply, your brain has turned to mush. Sound familiar? I hear it all the time from clients in diet mode, who are eating fewer calories and/or eliminating food groups.

I tell them that this forgetfulness and confusion isn't their fault. It's simple cause and effect: when you restrict the amount of fuel your brain has to work with, your brain is going to sputter. Especially if you restrict the healthy complex carbohydrates found in fruits, vegetables, and whole grains or are on a low-fat diet. (The brain needs fat to stabilize.)

The body breaks carbohydrates into a simple sugar called glucose, the brain's primary source of fuel. Because brain cells cannot store glucose, they depend on the bloodstream to deliver a constant supply.[15] In fact, Roy Baumeister and John Tierney note in their book *Willpower* that glucose is necessary for exerting self-control. Dieting tends to deplete glucose, which accounts for why it's so hard to forgo extra treats. In fact, this led to the idea that drinking orange juice, which provides glucose to the brain, can actually help you exert more self-control.

In a 2009 study conducted at Tufts University,[16] researchers had nineteen women follow one of two weight-loss diets: either a low-carb plan or a low-calorie plan that included complex carbohydrates.

The researchers had the low-carb group consume zero grams of carbs per day in week one, five to eight grams per day in week two, and ten to sixteen grams per day in week three. (That's truly a low-carb plan!) The women in the low-calorie group were instructed to calculate their daily calories based on their current weight and to choose foods on the Academy of Nutrition and Dietetics' food exchange lists. While this study

diet containing both sufficient calories and ample amounts of nutrients (see www.nutrition.org.uk for the British Nutrition Foundation advice or www.eatforhealth.gov.au if you live in Australia). Without good nutrition, it's hard to stay positive and optimistic—a key skill in emotional intelligence.

didn't report what the groups ate, a review of both groups' food journals found that the low-carb group was 93.3 percent in compliance with its guidelines, while the low-calorie group was 90.5 percent in compliance.

Before the women began the plans, the researchers gave them a series of tests used to measure long-term memory, short-term memory, and attention. Once the plans began, the tests were repeated weekly.

Remember, the women on the low-carb plan consumed zero carbohydrates during their first week on their plan. In tests given after week one, the low-carbers performed more poorly on memory-based tasks than the women on the low-calorie plan.

Also, compared to the low-calorie group, they had slower reaction times, and their visual-spatial memories (including the ability to judge distances, assemble a puzzle, and other tasks) were not as sharp. In tests given *after* week one, when small amounts of carbs had been added back to their diets, the low-carbers' performance on memory tests improved.

Dieting may also affect memory, an Australian study of thirty-two female dieters suggests.[17] In part, that may be because when your mind is preoccupied with thoughts of food, it can be hard to remember important stuff (or even simple stuff, like where you put your keys).

In Eat.Q. mode, it's important to consume the number of calories your brain and body need to function at their peak. That number is determined by your age, gender, and activity level. (To find expert-recommended guidelines, UK-based readers should visit www.nutrition.org.uk, the website of the British Nutrition Foundation. If you are based in Australia, visit www.eatforhealth.gov.au.)

Using Eat.Q. to Solve Eating Dilemmas

Can't stop munching? Feel like giving up? Tap into EI and Eat.Q., which can help you solve these and other common eating dilemmas.

| You want to stop munching but find it difficult to do so even though you know you've had enough. | Use: *Impulse Control*
To shift from "munch" to "stop," it can be helpful to imagine a car decelerating from 60 mph to a full stop.
1. Imagine driving in your car, looking at your speedometer.
2. Holding that image, ease your foot off the accelerator until the car comes to a full stop.
3. Now, mimic that deceleration as you "coast" to a full stop with your munching. Reach into your bag of crisps more slowly (one reach every minute, then every two minutes, and so forth), or add time (one minute, two minutes) between each crisp. |
| You experience the what-the-hell effect. | Use: *Flexibility*
When you notice black-and-white thinking, such as *I blew it—I'm going to eat as much as I want,* or *I can't eat anything until 6:00 P.M.,* use yoga thinking—that is, stretch your options. Let's say you want a milk shake. Here's how you employ yoga thinking:
1. Find the two extreme end points of your decision. Typically, these might be "I can have this milk shake" or "I cannot have this milk shake."
2. Imagine those two end points on a line—one at the beginning of the line, and one at the end.
3. Find the middle point on that line ("I can drink half the milk shake").
4. Identify other possible points (say, "I can drink two-thirds of the milk shake"). Finding these other possible end points helps remind you that you have more options than simply "I can have it all" or "I can't have it at all." |

You feel like you need a healthy eating plan but are not sure which one to pick.	Use: *Self-Awareness* There are so many healthy eating plans that include a wide variety of foods, you may not know which one fits your unique preferences. To identify the plan that complements your personality, tap into your self-awareness.

1. Create a list of the foods that you love and enjoy.
2. Now, write another list of foods that aren't as important to you.
3. Review the list. Notice any patterns? If you love chicken, being a vegetarian obviously won't work for you. On the other hand, if you enjoy fish, a Mediterranean style of eating may appeal. Dismiss any plans that work against the food lists you created above.
4. If you're still not sure which plan to choose, or if you have health concerns, ask a professional dietician or your doctor for suggestions.

You want to give up.	Use: *Motivation* Positive self-talk can help you carry on in the face of difficult change. If you notice that your self-talk is negative ("This stinks! I can't do it!"), begin to practice self-talk that focuses on *resilience,* the ability to bounce back from and cope with adversity.

1. Recall other significant changes you've made in your life. Did you quit smoking? Stick to an exercise program for a long period of time? End a relationship that wasn't working for you?
2. To build your resilience, engage in a few minutes of positive self-talk every day, especially around mealtimes. Examples of positive self-talk include:
   I can do this.
   Change is hard, but possible.
   I've done harder things than this.

Changing your diet makes you cranky (your mind says, *It's not fair!*)	Use: *Optimism* Changing the way you eat is never easy, but it's essential to remain hopeful that change is possible. If you don't think anything will change, nothing will! To build optimism, try visualization. 1. Find a quiet moment, or make one. 2. Close your eyes and "see" yourself living the changes you want to make. For example, you might visualize yourself taking one cookie from the box, closing the box, putting the box back in the cupboard, and walking away with confidence. 3. Repeat several times a day, especially when you're feeling cranky or blue. Implanting these images into your memory can help you trick your brain. The image in your brain tells it that you have done this before (even though it was imagined) and will make actions easier to do in the future.
You want a small piece but aren't sure what "small" really looks like.	Use: *Self-Regulation* Eat mindfully—that is, slowly, savoring each bite and using all of your senses. We'll discuss mindful eating more fully in the next few chapters.
You tend to eat more when you dine with other people.	Use: *Social Skills* 1. Lose the diet talk. It's no fun to eat with people who are chatting about their latest diet. Also, it pushes your companions to promote black-and-white thinking—"Oh, live a little and have dessert. We're having a good time." 2. Join with others on the topic of healthy eating. Talk about organic foods, cooking, and great restaurants. This minor shift in language will help to reset group norms (a shift from discussing what you can't eat to what you can eat). They say that the best way to learn something is to teach it. Therefore, find a pupil and get to work!

The Last Bite

If you've lived in diet mode for most of your life, I can understand how difficult it is to let go of the hope that the next diet will be the one that "works." I also understand that it may feel strange to let go of what may seem to you like dieting "gospel"—counting calories, using willpower, and so forth. As you read this chapter, did your mind rebel, or are you rethinking the whole concept of dieting? At this point in the book, it's a good time to open your mind and embrace a new approach to food, eating, and weight management—the Eat.Q. approach. I often share a Mark Twain quote with my clients because it sums up the way dieting becomes an emotional hurdle: "To promise not to do a thing is the surest way in the world to make a body want to go and do that very thing." This fits the bill with dieting. Forbidding yourself is a recipe for driving you further from, not closer to, your goals.

In the next chapter, we'll explore the delightful—and challenging—hurdles presented by pleasure eating.

5

Pleasure Seeking

Tell me what you eat, and I will tell you what you are.

—Jean Anthelme Brillat-Savarin

In 1825, an extraordinary book took the culinary capital of the world, Paris, by storm. Today that book, *The Physiology of Taste: Or, Meditations on Transcendental Gastronomy*[1], is still required reading for people who love to cook and eat. This witty collection of recipes, history, philosophy, and personal reflections has been in print for more than two hundred years.

Although he's considered one of the founding fathers of gastronomy, Jean Anthelme Brillat-Savarin wasn't a chef but a lawyer and politician from the town of Belley. (How perfect!) His genius lay not in preparing food but in celebrating it.

food for THOUGHT

- Is eating an event for you—something special—or a routine, akin to brushing your teeth?
- Is the pleasure you derive from food a matter of quantity or quality?
- Are your food selections typically driven by a desire to experience pleasure or to satisfy hunger?
- Do you typically choose real food that pleases your eye, delights your palate, and nourishes your body?
- Does pleasurable food make you feel out of control? Does your desire for pleasure when you eat outweigh every other consideration?

And good food *is* to be celebrated, is celebration itself—the Sunday dinner, the church supper, the holiday or birthday celebration, the brunch with friends. Often we derive as much pleasure from gathering around a table with friends and family as from the food itself.

But I wonder what Brillat-Savarin would say about the pleasure of eating if he were alive today. Eating is as necessary to life as drawing breath. But now that we don't have to hunt or gather food—now that it's a phone call or drive away—we rarely experience the pleasure of satisfying true physical hunger. Eating is no longer an event to be savored but a habit we indulge in around the clock.

My hope for all my clients, and for you, is that you recapture the pleasure Brillat-Savarin wrote about: pleasure rooted neither in denial nor overindulgence but in conscious appreciation—when you balance pleasure with mindful choice. In this chapter, you'll learn what kind of pleasure eater you are. You'll also learn why you take part in pleasure-based eating, when you're making pleasure-driven decisions to eat, and how to tame the need for pleasure eating in a world that pushes us toward it.

Much of Brillat-Savarin's advice on how to enjoy good food sensibly still rings true today. For example, expounding upon the dangers of taking too much pleasure in food, then known by the term *gourmandise,* he declared, "Gourmandise is an act of judgment."

Yes! When it comes to food, your experience of pleasure is rooted in how you define it and the decisions you make based on that definition. What researchers have added to Brillat-Savarin's intuitive understanding of pleasure eating is an understanding of exactly how that judgment begins in our brains—how the brain interacts with our senses to make decisions. As you'll see, pleasure isn't easy for the brain to resist. But when you use your emotional intelligence and a mindful pause, you can cool your need for instant gratification and weigh short-term pleasure against a long-term solution.

This Is Your Brain in a Fast-Food Nation

To us, pleasure is a value meal or a slice of banana cream pie. To neuroscientists, it's the brain's "like" reaction, conscious or no, to a reward—burger, pie, sex, illicit drugs, video games. They have discovered hedonic hot spots and circuits within the brain (hedonic from the Greek *hedone,* meaning "pleasure"). When stimulated by pleasurable stimuli, including food, they light up like slot machines in Las Vegas.[2]

Even this basic explanation of how the brain generates pleasure—by no means fully understood—suggests that while the human brain is a wondrous, elegant machine, it's no match for our society's constant cues to eat.

To live in the West is to be inundated with these cues. Doughnut and coffee shops, fast-food chains, and pizza places are part of the landscape. We live in what researchers call a *toxic food environment*—unhealthy food everywhere, available at any time, and constant media messages to relax, let go, *indulge*.

While the biology of sensory pleasure is beyond the scope of this book, to learn even the basics of how the brain responds to pleasure leads to one conclusion: in our food-centric society, it's extraordinarily difficult—a feat, in fact—to respond mindfully to the urge for pleasure.

A study in the *Journal of the American Dietetic Association* views overeating as a result of ways the brain controls eating behavior in response to environmental cues.[3] Even smart, highly motivated people struggle to not eat the dazzling array of intensely tasty foods high in sugar, salt, and fat available around the clock, the study found. The authors of the study identified three neurobehavioral processes implicated in overeating:

Food Reward. Largely regulated by a pathway in the brain called the mesolimbic dopamine system (aka "the reward circuit"), the food reward process includes both the experience of pleasure from eating and the motivational drive to get and eat highly palatable foods. Those with greater sensitivity to reward have stronger food cravings for sweet and fatty foods. Coupled with easy access to food, this biologically based sensitivity makes you highly vulnerable to overeating and weight gain.

Inhibitory Control. The brain's prefrontal cortex, which governs self-control, planning, and goal-directed behavior, is largely responsible for saying no despite a strong motivation to eat. Research suggests that a specific part of the prefrontal cortex, called the dorsolateral region, seems to help you "put on the brakes" and choose a salad instead of fries, or eat one serving of ice cream and stop.

Time Discounting. Humans typically value rewards given *now*. So, given a choice between an immediate "reward" (ice cream!) over losing a pound this week, we'll typically choose the ice cream. The link between time

WHAT IS PLEASURE?

Whether you're savoring your favorite ice cream, making love, or wandering around a museum, you experience *pleasure*. It's a kaleidoscope of a word, used to describe a wide array of positive mental states—enjoyment, fulfillment, ecstasy—that we humans deem worthy of seeking out.

What's fascinating is that it's not the ice cream, partner, or painting that holds the pleasure. Rather, research suggests that specific parts of the brain paint a "gloss" onto the sensation it elicits so that you "like" it, whether or not you're consciously aware of it.[4]

In psychology, the *pleasure principle* describes pleasure as a positive feedback mechanism that motivates us (and all animals) to recreate in the future a situation we have perceived as pleasurable in the past. (According to this theory, pioneered by Sigmund Freud, organisms are similarly motivated to avoid situations that have caused pain in the past.)

The experience of pleasure is subjective. In a given situation you, I, and a stranger will each experience varying kinds and amounts of pleasure, or none at all. Some stimuli are more likely to elicit pleasure than others, however. It's thought that pleasure helps fulfill Darwinian imperatives of survival and procreation. In other words, we have sex because it feels good, but it also results in furthering the species. Thankfully, it also feels good to eat, which is needed for survival.

Of course, some pleasures are less than healthy. For example, some drugs create euphoria in the brain. The natural tendency is to seek out more of this feeling, which can lead to dependence and addiction.

That being said, pleasure—which includes delight in good food—is essential to our well-being. However, don't mistake this particular pleasure with a food craving. A craving is an intense desire for a particular food. You don't want crisps or chocolate. You want barbecue-flavor crisps or a chocolate doughnut from the bakery around the corner from where you work, and nothing else will satisfy. By contrast, the desire to eat pleasurable foods means that you're human. The EAT method can help you manage that desire, so that you can experience pleasure *and* satisfy physical hunger.

discounting and body weight is governed by the reward system and the prefrontal cortex—the same region associated with the other two processes.

EI, Pleasure, and the PAUSE

Believe it or not, in Chicago, New York, and Los Angeles you can walk up to an ATM-like machine on the street and buy a cupcake.[5] Think about that for a moment. We live in a world where the cupcakes can come to you twenty-four hours a day. How can EI possibly help?

The answer is found in that sneaky trick Walter Mischel played on those marshmallow-loving four-year-olds. Numerous subsequent studies of the same four-year-olds who took part in the original study suggest that good things come to those who wait.

In the first follow-up, conducted fourteen years after Mischel's study, the kids who'd kicked tables and sung to themselves rather than eat the marshmallow when Mischel left were described by their parents as having significantly better emotional coping skills than those who'd gobbled the marshmallow immediately. A second follow-up, published in 1990, linked that ability to delay gratification and utilize self-control with higher SAT scores. Yet another, published in 2000—twenty-eight years after the original study—found that the marshmallow resisters had a higher sense of self-worth and a better ability to cope with stress.[6]

In 2012, there was yet another follow-up study published in the *Journal of Pediatrics*.[7] This one found that the kids who waited to eat their marshmallows now had a lower BMI than the marshmallow gobblers. For each minute they had refrained from reaching for the marshmallow, their BMI decreased 0.02 percent. So, by now you get it: impulse control is a good thing! It's exactly what you need to manage your world.

While you will never see the phrase "mindful pause" in Mischel's original study, you can see similarities between this strategy and those the kids were taught to help them refrain from eating the marshmallow. For example, Mischel told them to imagine the treat was just a picture with an imaginary frame around it, to reduce the children's focus on the sensory pleasure and disengage the part of the brain that anticipates food. He also instructed them to imagine that it was a cloud. Imagining that you're tasting a cloud, a non-food object not known to taste sweet, deflates the power of the craving.

Because instant gratification is built into modern life, it's hard to take the time to practice self-control. However, self-control is really just a "strategic allocation of your attention," to use Mischel's words. There's a big difference between suppressing your thoughts about a food you want and strategically allocating your attention. In thought suppression, you tell yourself, *Don't think about pizza!* or *I will not eat that brownie!*—a tactic research has shown just doesn't work. When you allocate your attention strategically, rather than not thinking about pizza, you change the *way* you think. (Mischel termed this *metacognition,* or thinking about your thinking process.) When you think about a food you crave, your mind starts to ponder how good it will taste, which increases your desire for it. Instead, try distracting yourself with the keep-calm tools in chapter 2 or any of the tools in chapter 10. Or think about your thoughts, such as *I'm really obsessing about pizza right*

PLAYING THE WAITING GAME

If four-year-olds can use mental tricks to delay gratification, so can you. For example, one of my clients told me she loves a certain type of biscuit—the bottoms are covered in chocolate while the tops are drizzled with horizontal chocolate stripes. It so happens that the stripes on the biscuit remind her of horizontal stripes on shirts, which she won't wear because she believes they make her look heavier. Thus, when she looks at the stripes on the biscuit, the mental association with stripes on a shirt immediately cools her desire. What a neat mental trick! I'm sure you can come up with similar transformations that work for you.

One of the best ways to learn to delay gratification—and thus increase your impulse control—is to build it into your daily routine. If you take the bus or the train to work, read your newspaper on your way home instead of on the way there. Or tackle your toughest task of the day first, and when you get it done, reward yourself with some mindless computer games (instead of playing the computer games first because, well, you want to). The more you practice delayed gratification, the easier it becomes to wait.

now. I wonder why. Either option is likely to work better than the just-say-no approach.

Eat.Q.: The Pursuit of Healthy Pleasure

One of my clients, Kelly, recently shared with me a story about her famous cherry-pineapple upside-down cake. When she brings this cake to work, it's gone within minutes.

One day, Kelly opened a coworker's office door to find that person licking the icing from the tinfoil that had covered the cake—she had confiscated and polished off the last few pieces. It's likely that the coworker's brain was surging with the feel-good brain chemical dopamine, released when you eat

> The next time you experience a craving, commit to not satisfying it for a set amount of time—try one to five minutes to begin with. In the early Mischel study, kids sang or played with a toy. Adult "distractions" include doing a crossword puzzle, composing and sending an e-mail, or cleaning out the kitchen junk drawer. (One caveat: before you begin your distraction, make sure there's no food within reach; you don't want to negate the power of the tool with mindless munching.) Okay? When you reach the five-minute time limit, decide to wait several more minutes—two, three, another five.
>
> If you're close to the food you crave (say, your partner's ice cream is in the freezer), take a page from Mischel's study: imagine the item you crave as a painting with a frame around it, to transform the food in your mind into "not food." And remember, you're not resisting a craving. You're engaging your mind in a "strategic allocation of your attention." In other words, you're focusing your mind away from the sensual pleasure you will obtain from food and instead focusing on thoughts that will help you wait.

sugary, fatty food. She had a hard time saying no (inhibitory control), as evidenced by the multiple slices and wanting it *now*.

I love this story. Who hasn't been that coworker? Even so, had Kelly's colleague used the EAT method she could have turned to a healthier way to get the pleasure she sought (or at least stopped at a single slice).

For example, Kelly used a mindful pause to help her perceive the first inkling of her urge for pleasurable food, which Kelly's coworker may have tuned out until it blindsided her. Perceiving pleasure can also mean get-

THE CASE OF THE SKYDIVING FOODIE

The pleasurable nature of food is transient: it comes and goes. Just as important, it changes. That's because the pleasure you derive from food is not necessarily inherent in the food itself but in your relationship with it.

That point was driven home for me after one of my clients, a wealthy, high-powered executive, suffered a skydiving accident. While he was fortunate to survive with bumps, bruises, and a broken arm, the accident knocked out several of his teeth and altered his jaw.

He didn't have PTSD, as I suspected he might after such an accident. In fact, he was ready to skydive again once his doctor gave him the all clear. But he appeared to be experiencing mild symptoms of depression.

Very quickly, his sessions began to focus on food. To my surprise, I noticed that we were talking a lot about the changes he experienced in his perception of pleasure. He had Brillat-Savarin's passion for good food. For this dedicated foodie, who sought out exquisite cuisine in high-end eateries, food wasn't a matter of nourishment, but pleasure. Overnight, his experience of food changed dramatically, hence the depression.

The pain limited what he could chew. For a time, he feared food—eating had become a source of pain rather than pleasure. He spoke at great lengths about the foods he missed, and he no longer wanted to make dinner dates with friends. ("What's the point? I won't enjoy it anyway.") He cared not a whit that he'd lost weight. Substantially over-

ting reacquainted with what foods (Ice cream? Cinnamon toast? Hummus? Steak?) give you pleasure.

Remember, it's okay to want food that gives you pleasure. (I wonder if Kelly's colleague knew that. My sense is that she didn't.) But it's also important to go the extra step: to discern what message wanting pleasurable food sends you about how you feel in the moment. Are you stressed? Bored? Unhappy? Relaxed? Take a moment to calm down and really think it through.

Once you have given your mind room to make a decision, when you raise

weight before his accident, he would have been risking his health if his pleasure-driven eating had continued.

One good result came from his ordeal. Unable to eat with the abandon he'd once had, he began to see how much eating had dominated his life and was forced to confront the fact that the majority of his eating had been pleasure-driven.

First, we had to work through the despair of loss—his primary source of pleasure had been ripped away. Then, we focused on discovering new sources of pleasure. As was clear by his newfound love of skydiving, he liked things that gave him an adrenaline rush, which may relate to why he liked food so much. Both flying through the air and eating an over-the-top dessert gave his senses an instant and short-term high.

Once his jaw healed, he tried to return to his favorite dishes and was shocked by how rich and heavy many were. To his surprise, he no longer enjoyed them. He developed a new pleasure in healthier foods—mashed sweet potatoes, gnocchi with chard and white beans, braised meats (easier on his jaw). While he still derived pleasure from food, he ate with more discernment. He had, from necessity, followed Brillat-Savarin's aphorism: eating had become an act of judgment.

My skydiving foodie taught me something, too: Our perceptions of pleasure aren't fixed. They can change based on our circumstances and new ways of thinking. In fact, if you feel that only certain foods can do it for you, you may be missing out.

your Eat.Q., sometimes you'll indulge in pleasurable food mindfully, and sometimes you'll pass it up. That's the perk of learning how to anticipate both short-term and long-term outcomes.

Those abilities will come, I promise. But for now, let's explore your deepest attitudes, feelings, and beliefs about whether it's okay to enjoy pleasurable foods. Ultimately, it comes down to three choices: denial, overindulgence, or finding and maintaining a healthy balance between the two.

THE EAT METHOD MODEL OF PLEASURE SEEKING

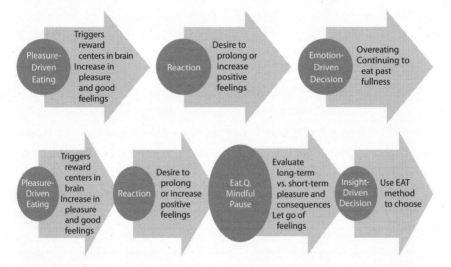

Pleasure-driven eating begins in the brain, but there can be too much of a good thing. When you take a mindful pause, you'll be able to slow down long enough to weigh short-term pleasure (tempting foods) against long-term goals (weight loss or maintenance).

Are You a Depriver, a Fiver, or a Take-Me-Higher?

Journalists often call me for tips on how to master emotional eating. One of their most common questions is "Is it okay to enjoy food and eating?" I give them a resounding *yes!* It's more than okay. In fact, it's necessary and part of learning to make insight-driven decisions.

To understand why, consider the following University of California, San Diego, study on chocolate, a food many people consider one of the most pleasurable foods on the planet.[8]

Analyzing the eating habits of nearly a thousand healthy adults, the researchers found that those who ate chocolate more than twice a week—the average consumption of the people studied—had a lower BMI than those who ate it less often. This despite the fact that the frequent chocolate eaters did not eat fewer calories (they actually ate more) or exercise more. Indeed, the researchers couldn't identify any behavioral differences that explained the finding.

The researchers concluded that the calories in chocolate may be offset by other ingredients that boost metabolism. Is their theory true? I don't know, and neither do they. But as I read the study, I had a theory of my own: might it be that the regular chocolate eaters were thinner because they have a more relaxed attitude toward eating—exactly the attitude that people with high Eat.Q.s display?

Adapting this study to mimic the type of pleasure eaters I tend to see in my office, I mentally grouped the participants (and people in general) into three categories:

The Deprivers. Those who are dieting, don't eat chocolate or pleasurable food, and fight their desire for the pleasurable food they crave. In the University of California study, this group had higher BMIs.

The Fivers. In the study, these people ate at least five pieces of chocolate a week. Fivers have learned to incorporate a food they like, such as chocolate, into their lives without diving headlong into overindulgence.

The Take-Me-Highers. These are the people who eat chocolate to excess. While not a category in the University of California study, it's known that a portion of the population overindulges in the sweet stuff. While "overindulgence" in chocolate is unique to each person, a reasonable working definition might be eating chocolate more than once a day. If I had to guess, I'd say it's likely that the people in this study who forbid themselves from overeating chocolate, and then overindulged, are emotional eaters. Criticism of the study said that the higher-weight volunteers may have not admitted to eating as much chocolate as they actually do. (Because it may not be socially acceptable to admit to eating lots of chocolate, they may have underreported how much chocolate they consume to look good.)[9] However, other research suggests that depriving yourself or trying to suppress thoughts of chocolate makes you crave it more.[10]

Which category do you fit in? Just as important is whether a more relaxed attitude about eating pleasurable food has an effect on your BMI.

People with high Eat.Q.s might be described as fivers. They can identify the need for pleasure in food and manage—even shape—that need, perhaps by taking their version of a mindful pause.

By contrast, those with few Eat.Q. skills have difficulty regulating pleasure-driven eating, either denying themselves (deprivers) or overindulging (take-me-highers). Either way, if you aren't mindful when you eat, the act of eating can easily turn into a stream of pleasure followed by displeasure. The more pleasurable food you eat, the more habituated you become to it, and the less pleasurable it seems to you. Or, conversely, the more of it you crave. (Research suggests that the brains of people who are overweight or obese react more intensely to food.)

QUIZ: DO YOU HIDE FROM PLEASURE OR SEEK IT?

Do you try to ignore the natural human need for pleasure, or do you feel ruled by it? How much does the pursuit of pleasure affect what you put on your plate? Take this simple quiz to find out.

1. You are on a deadline and must turn in a project by tomorrow at 8:00 A.M. It's time for dinner and you're starving. You . . .

   a. skip dinner—no time to eat.

   b. nuke a hot dog or grab a handful of crackers or pretzels. You just need something to tide you over, and anything will do.

   c. heat up leftovers and munch a brownie while you work.

   d. set aside your project and order something sumptuous. Or cook— there's always time to chop vegetables for a salad or simmer a sauce. Hey, you can't be creative if you don't enjoy your meal.

2. When you have a craving you . . .

   a. ignore it.

   b. satisfy it and move on.

   c. obsess about it, cave in, satisfy it, and eat more of it than you wanted to.

   d. not only indulge it, but continue to eat it. Sometimes you can't stop.

3. As you walk into a bakery to buy bread, the baker is pulling out
    a tray of cinnamon rolls, your all-time favorite. Which thought is
    likely to talk you into eating it?

    a. No way. You're on a diet.

    b. They smell heavenly. And that gooey icing on a fresh-from-the-
        oven bun will just melt in your mouth.

    c. Why not? Just one. You'll really enjoy it.

    d. There is no thought when it comes to cinnamon buns. You leave
        with a bag full of them and eat until you feel ill.

4. You tend to seek a pleasure food . . .

    a. rarely. As long as you're not hungry, you're fine.

    b. occasionally. You like a few particular things but won't go out of
        your way to enjoy them. Besides, they're too expensive.

    c. a few times a week. If you notice you're craving a food you love,
        you seek it out.

    d. constantly. You need something yummy at every meal and snack.

5. For you, chocolate is . . .

    a. not important. You don't eat it or many sweet things.

    b. a semi-annual indulgence. You eat it on holidays and birthdays,
        but otherwise you can take it or leave it.

    c. a necessity of life. You buy a bag or box of your favorites, which
        lasts a month or so, and keep it for indulgent moments.

    d. kryptonite—your only natural weakness. Once you taste it, it's
        off to the races.

6. If you want a snack, you seek something . . .

    a. close at hand. To satisfy your hunger, you'll grab whatever.

    b. healthy and quick. Carrot sticks or a plain granola bar.

    c. satisfying. But not chocolate; you know it will trigger cravings.

    d. chocolaty, salty, or fatty—stuff that makes your taste buds tap
        dance.

7. You're most likely to seek pleasurable food when you're . . .

    a. You don't. You know splurging on your favorite food will make you feel incredibly guilty.

    b. frustrated. You start to roam the kitchen, opening and shutting the refrigerator or cupboards.

    c. in a certain mood, such as stressed out. Pleasurable food gives you a quick pick-me-up.

    d. awake. Just about any mood can make you want something rich and delicious.

8. Imagine you're ordering from a menu. List the following in order of importance:

    a. Health. A food may taste great, but really you're looking at the most nutritious option.

    b. Amount or portion size. You like to feel full.

    c. Overall satisfaction—how filling and pleasing the dish will be to your palate.

    d. Taste. You prefer amazing, complex flavors, no matter how many calories.

SCORING

Give yourself zero points for each (a) answer, one point for each (b) answer, two points for each (c) answer, and three points for each (d) answer.

0–8 points: Depriver. You have a utilitarian view of eating, but could you be hiding from pleasure? It may be that your task is to enjoy food in a meaningful and thoughtful way. Not caring about what you eat may be as dangerous as caring too much. You're not likely to find a balance or put in any effort if you just don't pay attention to food.

9–16 points: Fiver. You welcome pleasure into your life and may be working on moderating it. This is often a delicate line to walk between honoring this need without overdoing it. Your challenge may be to continue to find that balance. The Eat.Q. approach will point you toward understanding what truly gives you pleasure and whether sensory tastes and emotions trigger your need for more pleasurable food or less.

17–24 points: Take-Me-Higher. You're a bona fide pleasure seeker. You may find that many of your decisions are dominated by a desire for foods that tantalize your taste buds, even if only in the short term. It's likely that you feel completely out of control when you're eating sweets and things that inherently taste good. If this sounds like you, your task is to turn to the tools in the T section (see chapter 11), which will help you moderate your eating.

Do You Eat in the Past, Present, or Future?

Which type of food from the following list most resonates with you?

a. A comfort food, such as your mum's famous casserole or real mashed potatoes with butter—the kind served with a holiday meal.

b. A food that's considered decadent, or one with complex flavors—pasta puttanesca; meat with a balsamic vinegar, brown sugar, and hot-pepper glaze; or dense chocolate cake layered with a delicate mousse filling and topped with fluffy whipped cream.

c. A meal at your favorite restaurant, one that you have to make reservations for in advance. You already know you love it. You're already beginning to visualize what from the menu you'll have. You might even daydream about the exact dish you'd order.

I ask this question because there's another way to reveal the role of pleasurable food in your life—whether you tend to eat in the past, present, or future. Once you truly tune in to why a particular food delights you, you can respond to that tug for pleasure in a mindful way.

Think of the foods you love. Do they share any common pleasurable elements—a certain taste (sweet, salty) or a particular texture (creamy, crunchy)? Are these foods linked to strong and specific memories? Or is the best part of any meal or snack planning what you're going to have?

Ponder your answer as you read the next few sections, which identify each type of pleasure eater—past, present, or future—and offer a customized tip.

The Blast-from-the-Past Eater

Your most pleasurable foods have a memory component—they evoke pleasurable experiences from your past. The memory of a food that felt good or comforting in the past is stored in the amygdala, the part of the brain that performs a primary role in the processing and memory of emotional reactions.

THE THREE-MINUTE CHOCOLATE FIX

I'm sure after a stressful day you've thought, *Chocolate would make me feel better.* You're right; chocolate does make us feel good . . . temporarily. But would you like to know how long that boost in mood lasts?

Three minutes. That's right—researchers clocked it. Furthermore, chocolate's ability to elevate mood depends on its quality.

In a study published in the journal *Appetite*,[11] 113 normal-weight volunteers, who were in a bad mood, were given different qualities of chocolate—good (considered tasty) and not so good. Only the good chocolate affected a negative mood. The researchers hypothesized that the palatable chocolate's brief positive effects on mood were due to the immediate sensory pleasure (the taste on the tongue) and the volunteers' emotional associations with chocolate (their blissful memories of chocolate). It's unlikely that the chocolate affected brain chemicals in three minutes. Generally speaking, any physiological change takes up to an hour.

The take-home message is that, if you're going to indulge in chocolate, I recommend you splurge on a small piece of the highest quality variety you can find—rich, dark "boutique" chocolate rather than cheap, mass-processed stuff. If the pleasure lasts only three minutes, then make the most of them!

A mum and professor at a small college, Emma struggled with her cravings. They seemed different from those her colleagues experienced. While they snuck sweets from the office or joked about how many biscuits they ate during the holiday break, her cravings seemed more elaborate. She couldn't understand why she couldn't lose weight. She didn't touch the sweets and was happy with one or two biscuits during the entire holiday season. Why did her cravings seem so different from theirs?

One day, in session, I asked her the *pleasure* question. After a moment, she said she liked foods that "stuck to her bones."

Hmm. "Did someone tell you that?" I asked. "Your mum or dad maybe?"

She smiled. "Yes." Mealtimes in her home were an event, not a daily task, she explained. She grew up with a mum always swaddled in an apron, and in a region, where chicken and dumplings and chard greens swimming in lard were standard fare.

Comfort foods tap into the emotional parts of the brain and your memory. For Emma, the foods she craved were an emotional connector to her past. Embodied in the dishes she made were the images, smells, and tastes imbued in her childhood. They transported her back to her mother, whom she missed dearly, and the pace and lifestyle of the south. She still felt out of place with her colleagues. Comfort foods seemed to call her name when she was stressed and—most important—feeling out of place.

TIP FOR BLAST-FROM-THE-PAST EATERS

When the need for a classic comfort food beckons, press PAUSE (page 47). Then, use the peek-behind-the-craving tool (page 55). Both can help you get in touch with what's prompting that need for a particular food. Is it caused by a specific feeling? Or a desire to reconnect with happy times long past? Or discomfort with a particular relationship or situation that makes you long for a happier, simpler time in your life?

Once you find your answer, sit with it for another full minute. Then, try a stress-reducing exercise, like one of the keep-calm tools in chapter 2.

Raising her Eat.Q. did not mean cutting these comfort foods from her life entirely. Chicken and dumplings was her taste of home, the *ahhh* in her soul. Her task was to tune herself to what triggered her desire for these foods. Understanding how these emotions popped up, rather than focusing on the specific foods she craved, made a significant difference. She began to recognize when her feeling-out-of-place button was pushed, so she could tune in to other sources of comfort and pleasure.

The Right-Here-Right-Now Eater

Your most pleasurable foods have a sensory component to them—not just flavor, but texture and contrasts too. When I asked Jonathan, a thirty-year-old equipment salesperson, what kind of food he liked, he had a very long list and definite specifications: crunchy, salty foods; particular types of sweets (black licorice); and combinations of hot and sweet (spicy barbecued spare ribs) and sweet and salty (sugared nuts). The taste of a dish came before anything else. He noticed he had become bored with food, particularly because he and his wife had gotten into a repetitive cycle of meals. Monday night spaghetti, Tuesday night steak, Wednesday night stir-fry . . . a few days of a bland, repetitive menu, and his taste buds were ripe for rebellion.

That's when he began craving foods that gave him a very high jolt—fast-food tacos, high-sugar cereals, stuffed-crust pizzas. Or he'd go to a local Indian restaurant for lamb curry, extra hot, with a side dish of cool, creamy cucumber-and-yogurt *raita*. The contrast between the two flavors and textures pleased him.

When he got frustrated with his weight, he tried diets. But the lackluster taste didn't do it for his thrill-seeking tongue. In fact, the more he ramped down the taste—oatmeal with no brown sugar, for example—the more intense his cravings for specific tastes became.

"Why do I go for this stuff?" he asked me. "I *know* it's not good for me. Why does everything always have to taste *amazing*?"

I suggested that he stop fighting against his tastes (and stop the dieting, too). We worked on getting to know his tastes well, identifying what foods he felt vulnerable around and finding creative ways to ramp up taste without ramping up calories. I remember sending him on a shopping expedition for

TIP FOR RIGHT-HERE-RIGHT-NOW EATERS

Like Jonathan, many of us experience *sensory-specific satiety,* which essentially means we tire of foods as we eat them. This is one reason that, after we take a few bites of one food, we turn to another. That switch gives us pleasure.

From a biological perspective, eating a variety of foods is important, because different foods contain different nutrients, all of which our bodies need to function at their peak. So, food boredom is useful: it drives us to a variety of foods so our bodies get the nutrients they need.

Sensory eaters don't focus as much on nutrients, of course; *sensation* is what they're after. If you're a sensory eater, don't restrict variety. Boredom will derail your efforts. To use sensory-specific satiety to your advantage, increase variety rather than calories. Treat yourself to fresh herbs when you cook. Grind your own spices. Treat yourself to small portions of intensely flavored foods, such as bittersweet chocolate or blue cheese. The more options you give yourself, particularly in a single meal, the more pleasure you will experience.[12] (This is true for Right-Here-Right-Nows, but if you eat in the past or the future, too much variety may lead you to overeat.)

Another tip: consider laying down your fork after savoring one or two delicious mouthfuls. At that point, you've achieved maximum pleasure—you could eat more, but you won't enjoy it more!

fresh herbs and spices, since he loved Indian food. He came in the next week, excited about the fresh dill and coriander he'd "discovered" in the produce aisle. Now, he cooks dinner once a week—Indian, Cuban, Caribbean—and his cravings are in check.

The Foodturistic Eater

Your most pleasurable foods have an anticipatory component to them—planning to eat a desired food or meal is part of the pleasure for you. A combination of the words *food* and *futuristic, foodturistic* is a word I and one of my

TIP FOR FOODTURISTIC EATERS

If you spend a lot of time focusing on what you'll eat and when, what hopes, dreams, and goals are you *not* thinking about? Have you always wanted to start a garden, join your town's historical society, or take a painting class? Turn your daydreaming toward activities and aspirations beyond your next meal.

Also, when you find yourself daydreaming about food, bring yourself back with the tuning-in-to-the-now meditation (page 52).

clients, Kristine, made up to explain her daydreaming about where, when, and how she was going to eat her next meal. At breakfast, foodturistic eaters think of what they want for lunch and maybe even dinner. They daydream about it. They *plan* for it. All this mental preparation is almost as pleasurable as eating the food or meal itself. Typically, when they finally get it, they'll eat more than they really want to prolong that pleasure.

"I just like food more than people," Kristine said in one early session, with a combination of defiance and sadness. I didn't think so, although I kept that to myself. Ultimately, our work together revealed that her daydreaming about future meals hid emotional holes she was trying to fill with food. She was lonely without any current prospects of dating. Nights were particularly hard—she would come home from an unfulfilling job and headed straight for her sofa and her laptop. Ultimately, she made a decision to try activities that she found interesting, enrolling in a glassblowing class at a local university (you can't eat while you're working with hot glass!), and make deeper connections with others to find non-food sources of pleasure.

Keeping Pleasure, Letting Go of Pain

As we've seen, our food decisions are driven by pleasure, which is not a bad thing. The key is to *manage* pleasure, so you get all of its joy with none of the pain or guilt. In the next few sections, I'll explain how to do just that, the EAT method way.

E: Embrace by Learning to Perceive Pleasure

I have an acquaintance who dislikes ice cream. Maybe you find this hard to believe. Or perhaps you feel the same way.

My point? When I talk about perceiving pleasure, I'm talking about the way *you* experience pleasure from food. Your idea of pleasurable food—smooth, sweet, creamy ice cream or crunchy, salty chips or warm, savory foods like mashed potatoes or macaroni and cheese—is as unique to you as your fingerprint. (Though my friend turns up her nose at ice cream, she is defenseless against all manner of salty snacks, especially cheese curls.)

Perceiving pleasure involves the tasks in this next section. I've given examples of what I mean, but as you open the door to perceiving pleasure, I encourage you to draw on your own experiences to answer the following four questions:

To what extent do you use food for pleasure?

Tune in to your desire for pleasurable food. Perhaps you don't dare think about the foods that comfort you or make you happy when you eat them. Perhaps you view them as "bad." Are you willing to consider that foods are neither good nor bad, to see a slice of cake as neither good nor evil but as one edible item among countless others?

Once you tune in to the need for pleasure when you eat, it's necessary to consider other factors, like health. If you love pork crackling, you must first see, then accept, that you love it. Once that's settled, you can work on managing cravings with the peek-behind-the-craving exercise on page 55.

Which foods for you are pure sensory nirvana?

Determine what foods give you pleasure. Once you're receptive to the idea that food can be pleasurable, you can turn to this question. Maybe it's sticky buns, buttery mashed potatoes or rice, or tomatoes still warm from the sun, drizzled with olive oil and topped with fresh basil. Talk about sensory pleasure! Such a contrast to my friend's cheese curls—pleasurable, certainly, but in a different way.

FOUR WAYS TO CONQUER IMPULSE EATING

1. *Focus on gains, rather than losses.* Focus on the positives of healthy eating (I'll fit into my pants) versus the negatives (I won't be able to fit into my current trousers). Fear doesn't motivate good decisions. In fact, we shy away from things we fear, including decisions, and are more likely to just give in.[13]

   Include in your "gains" the benefits you reap *right now*. Making beneficial decisions about your future health doesn't often win out over your current happiness. As humans, we naturally lean toward short-term rather than long-term pleasure. So, take a moment to think about or jot down a list of what you gain now, in this moment, when you pass up a second slice of pie (peace of mind, a lack of guilt, a lack of feeling too full, a satisfied feeling).

2. *Use stop signs.* A study in *Behaviour Research and Therapy* found that placing an actual stop sign near tempting food led to a decrease in choosing palatable foods while increasing the subjects' choices of healthy foods.[14] The researchers indicated that the stop signals (the color red) increased healthy decisions because it helped to slow down automatic impulses. (If you don't have stop signs, red plates or napkins can play the same function—seeing red makes you stop!)

3. *When in doubt, chill out.* The common wisdom is that, to withstand temptation, we need to take action—"exert" willpower, "fight" temptation, "control" desires. However, a 2012 study published in the journal *Motivation and Emotion* found that volunteers primed with "passive" words such as *rest, stop,* or *relax* were less likely to make impulsive decisions.[15] By contrast,

volunteers primed to use "action" words had poorer impulse control than those primed with the passive words. The study noted that passive words have been shown to have a relaxing effect on people and that the relaxed state better inhibits the pull of temptation.

The take-home message is that, when the impulse to eat hits, use passive words. For example, the next time you're hit with an urge to open the freezer for some ice cream, tell yourself, *Just relax and hang out on the sofa. No need to get up.*

4. *Reset your expectations.* People in emotional distress tend to impulsively eat more comfort foods and unhealthy snacks because they believe it makes them feel better, makes them happier, or repairs their mood.[16] Expectations are powerful. It's easy to keep eating in hope that the feeling you're waiting for will eventually come.

   But what if you reset your expectations as to what food can realistically deliver, such as relief from hunger and fleeting pleasure? I tell my clients to first listen closely to their thoughts to understand their expectations—what do they *think* they will feel? You can use this information, too. Listen for phrases like: *I* need *this brownie. It will make me feel better.* If you hear this in your mind, give yourself a gentle mental nudge. Remind yourself that food doesn't come with a money-back guarantee if it doesn't deliver comfort. Say to yourself, *I only* think *this brownie will help, but in ten minutes I'll feel yucky again.* Then, choose an alternative to the brownie that *does* make you feel good for the long term, such as a soothing cup of tea or flipping through a magazine.

Are you a past, present, or future pleasure eater?

Diagnose your need for pleasure. Do your food choices evoke memories of past pleasure from comfort foods, offer present sensual pleasure, or prolong into the future the pleasure you seek or are experiencing?

When do you find yourself needing pleasurable foods most?

Become aware of making decisions based on your desire for pleasure. You've discovered that sometimes (often?) you want food to be a delight to eat. Otherwise, you'd contentedly munch nothing but bran flakes, cottage cheese, and grilled chicken breast. But now that you know which foods send you to the moon, make the connection. Sometimes you decide to eat certain foods knowing they will relax you, soothe you, make you *feel good*. You want pleasure, and these foods offer it.

Plus, ponder the factors that affect your decisions. Perhaps today you ate a fistful of chocolate-covered pretzels, your absolute favorite treat. Or a can of spaghetti hoops. (I have a friend whose husband, at fifty years old, enjoys them every few months.) What were you feeling in the moment you chose to eat that treat? Were you in a celebratory mood, angry at your spouse, feeling blue on a cold winter day? Or did you eat it because, like the mountain, it was there?

These questions matter. To raise your Eat.Q., you must learn to ask them and pause long enough to arrive at answers.

THE FOUR S'S OF PLEASURE EATING

When you fully enjoy food, you can feel better about eating less of it. The four S's can help.

1. *Sit.* It sounds simple: sit down. Avoid multitasking or walking around while you eat. Focus on your plate.

2. *Shift* into the moment. Take a deep breath. Take a close look before you dive into your plate. Appreciate the presentation of the food. How does it look to you? Like a piece of artwork? A mess dumped out of a fast-food bag?

3. *Sense.* Take note of your senses. How does your food look, smell, sound, taste, and feel to your touch? Notice the sound of chewing or the sizzle of meat. Take a whiff of the aroma. Roll around the bite in your mouth. Evaluate the spices and texture (creamy, crunchy, gooey).

4. *Savor.* Don't gulp, sip. Ramp down your speed. Sometimes it's easier said than done, but it's possible. Remind yourself, *Pace. Don't race.*

Fast Food: The "I Hate Myself for Loving You" Syndrome

Fast food tends to elicit strong feelings in people. They love it, hate it, or hate that they love it. This includes a former client of mine, Melanie.

A single mum and nurse in a busy pediatricians' practice, Melanie sought my help for stress eating; like many of my clients, she battled with her weight. Early on, I noticed that she had a particular distain for fast food. "I see its consequences every day at work—not just the parents, but the kids," she said. She lectured her own children on its evils and, in front of the TV at night, made sneering comments during fast-food commercials. In session, she went on fast-food diatribes.

Her behavior reminded me of the Shakespeare quote "Thou doth protest too much." But we continued to work on her stress eating.

However, in session one day she broke down: she *did* eat fast food. "Bacon cheeseburgers," she admitted, "after really stressful days at work." She described the first bite as "like an out-of-body experience."

She felt like a hypocrite, lecturing her kids about it. "Why do I eat this crap?" she said. "I never ate it as a kid."

Ah. "Never?" I asked.

"Never," Melanie replied. "My parents ate organic, mostly. They called fast food 'that crap.'"

I looked at her and raised my eyebrows. Time to activate EAT.

This is what we found: Melanie knew she ate when stressed, and her job offered a constant supply. Her office was chronically overbooked, yet she had to be calm and courteous in a crush of squalling babies, vomiting toddlers, and harried parents.

Breakthrough! Melanie noticed that her desire for fatty, bacon-y pleasure tended to pop up when her balky computer froze or shut down, as it did several times a day, leaving her unable to make appointments or process insurance claims for the harried parents in front of her. Her sense of powerlessness in this situation sent her over the edge. That's when the urge for a cheeseburger overwhelmed her, and she made the emotion-driven decision to satisfy it (*I deserve it!*).

Melanie had a lot of accepting to do. Together, I helped her accept that her parents' negativity toward fast food influenced her own, that her computer malfunctions were simply life, and that she *liked* bacon cheeseburgers and that was okay.

Once Melanie made those connections, she could accept her feelings of powerlessness and frustration, and her urge for pleasurable food and the emotions that triggered it, for what they were: an SOS from within. How would she respond?

We decided that when she got that SOS, she'd get up from her chair, no matter how frantic the office was, go to the ladies' room for at least two minutes, and do deep breathing or repeat a positive affirmation she'd chosen: "This, too, shall pass." She also decided to start a small indoor herb garden at home, to encourage her to cook healthy meals for herself and her kids. And if she *still* wanted the burger, she made the *intentional* decision to splurge, ordering the children's portion and eating it mindfully (see page 240).

What's the lesson here? The next time you're struggling against your desire for the number six at your favorite fast-food chain, press PAUSE. Without emotion, trace the source of your desire for *this* food, at *this* moment, to its source. It's likely that what you discover can help you make a conscious decision to answer the call to pleasure and hit the drive-through, or drive on by.

A: Accept and Use Your Pleasure-Food Triggers

Cravings for pleasurable food can be either scary or annoying. You don't want to think about them or decide what to do about them. You just want them to go away.

I understand. When you feel out of control around food—cornered by it—it's natural to try to wrest back that control. Perhaps, in your view, to regain control is to deny pleasure. It feels wrong, somehow, to desire the thing that holds you hostage.

However, *everyone* craves pleasurable foods, even people who don't struggle with food or their weight. In a food-centric society, food cravings are a fact of life, and it's not a matter of if you cave, but when. That said, you can control the way you respond to food cravings.

I've worked with enough eating-disordered clients to know that if you deny or resist your need for pleasurable food, you may win . . . for a time. But inevitably, you will experience a rebound effect and eat more than if you'd accepted that you were having a chocolate moment and indulged sensibly.

Several studies suggest as much. One review on the effect of chocolate on mood, published in the *Journal of Affective Disorders,*[17] notes that when you eat chocolate to satisfy a craving, you don't crave it anymore. But when you eat it to comfort yourself, it's more likely to prolong rather than end a blue mood. In another study published in the journal *Appetite,*[18] women who suppressed thoughts of a craved food—in this instance, chocolate—simply ate more of it when they gave in.

In this study, the researchers divided 116 young women into three groups. They instructed one group to not think about chocolate, one group to think about anything they wanted, and the last group to think specifically about chocolate. The don't-think-about-it group ate 50 percent more when offered it compared with the women who were told to think about chocolate.

However futile it may be, it's brave to try to resist pleasure. But it's equally courageous, and more effective, to transform resistance into acceptance—to confront it head-on so you can calmly determine where it's coming from and consciously decide to indulge or to pass it up this time. As you raise your Eat.Q., you'll see that it's possible to allow the human need for pleasure to be part of the experience of eating without it dominating your every choice.

PRACTICE BOOSTING YOUR EAT.Q. . . .
WITH ICE CREAM

This is not a diet book, and we all deserve the pleasure of ice cream now and then. The next time you indulge, try one or more of these tips to become more aware of the ways you experience gustatory pleasure:

Go for a cone. Kay McMath, a food technologist for New Zealand's Massey University, says a cone beats a dish for several reasons. Licking coats your tongue with a thin layer of ice cream, so it's more quickly warmed and the flavor is more rapidly detected by the taste buds. Spoons, on the other hand, keep ice cream colder longer, which means the ice cream doesn't release its flavor as fast. Also, when you lick a cone, you're getting a smaller amount than you would in a spoonful, so the full melt and flavor is released with every lick. Don't like the taste of cones, or don't want the extra calories? Think of it as a dish, and throw it away when you finish the ice cream.

The next time you order a cone, ask for a spoon too. Take a lick, then a spoonful. Notice any differences in flavor and satisfaction.

Use your powers of observation. What does your cone-eating "style" reveal about who you are and how you feel about pleasure? Do you do the straight lick or bite off chunks? Do you methodically eat off the sprinkles first? How do you feel if ice cream dribbles down your wrist—panicky? Delighted, like a five-year-old?

Freeze your eating speed. If you tend to eat too quickly, consider "brain freeze," the blinding headache that results when cold materials, such as ice cream or cold drinks, hit the warm roof of your mouth. Area blood vessels constrict to reduce the loss of body heat, then relax and allow blood flow to increase. The resulting burst of pain is the reason you learned early on not to gobble ice cream. The next time you eat a meal or snack, pretend you're eating an ice cream cone to practice eating more slowly.

T: Turn to Positively Managing Your Pleasure Foods by Working Them into Your Diet

Earlier in the chapter, I discussed a study that found that people who ate chocolate regularly were thinner than both those who deprived themselves and those who ate it constantly. Note the difference between regularly and constantly. The former implies breaks from pleasure; pleasure has its place in a fiver's diet but does not dominate it.

And so we arrive at the T of the EAT method—the *turning to*. In this case, the positive alternative is to work pleasurable foods into your diet so you can manage how often you eat them and how much of them you eat.

Working them in does not mean eating them every time you want to. Sometimes you decide to indulge, and sometimes you focus on future benefits, such as health or weight loss. The following exercise—which I've dubbed the marshmallow method in honor of Mischel's marshmallow study—can help you delay the impulse to eat a pleasurable food. Use it not to avoid the food you crave but to decide whether to indulge.

The Marshmallow Method

Should you snack on yogurt or a doughnut? Splurge on more pasta and garlic bread or stop? When you're in danger of letting your desire for pleasure make the decision for you, follow these steps:

1. Do a mindful pause. You need that pause to note that you've arrived at a moment of decision. Appreciate that you can't control whether you will lose weight in the future. *This* moment is the one you can control. *This* moment of decision is the one that matters.

2. Set a timer for five minutes.

3. Direct your thoughts away from how good that pleasurable food would taste and toward a neutral topic or activity. The kids in Mischel's study sang and counted to distract themselves. You can distract yourself in grown-up ways. Send an e-mail. Wash your kitchen floor. Paint your toenails. Count the books on your bookshelf or the tiles on your ceiling.

4. If waiting seems impossible, put a different frame around the craved food. Imagining whipped-cream frosting as shaving cream has a way of cooling desire.

5. When the buzzer rings make your decision. You have three options: eat the pleasurable food, eat some, or eat none. Choose one, and don't look back. Even if you've chosen to eat it, or eat some, you've still make an insight-driven decision rather than an emotion-driven one.

The Last Bite

Food can be one of life's greatest pleasures. But perhaps it's more accurate to say that to attain peak pleasure from food it's essential to balance the pleasure of eating with health and well-being. That balance is rooted in *mindful* eating. It's not always easy to find that balance, but the EAT method can help you temper your drive for pleasurable food. The formula is common sense: acknowledge your need for pleasure, stay a step ahead of your emotional triggers, and turn to tools that help temper your impulse to overindulge.

The late Julia Child—arguably the first real celebrity chef—knew a lot about finding pleasure in the kitchen and once famously said, "How can a nation be called great if its bread tastes like Kleenex?" I'd like to expand on this: How can *you* be called great if you eat bread that tastes like Kleenex? To be "great" is to learn the art of eating food that's both healthy *and* pleasurable, and in a mindful way.

In the next chapter, we'll explore the next barrier to a high Eat.Q.: social eating.

6

Social Eating

If you want to learn how other people truly affect the way you eat, share a meal in another country.

Several years ago, I traveled to Perugia, the capital city of the region of Umbria in central Italy, near the Tiber River. The mountain-ringed city is also world-renowned for its chocolate.

Once in the city, I met an old friend who took me home to dinner. A winding road brought us to her house, small but warm, nestled against terraces that overlooked the mountainside. The door flew open, and I saw a flash of white teeth and curly hair and heard a burst of Italian—my friend's

food for THOUGHT

- Do you eat more when you are alone, or when you eat with others?
- Do you have people in your life who hinder your efforts to eat well? How about people who support your efforts?
- Do you eat more when you're with a specific person, or in a specific situation?
- Do you eat more at home, at restaurants, or at parties?
- Do your feelings about yourself and your relationships determine what you put on your plate?

mother. Though this was our first meeting, she hugged me tightly, squeezing the breath out of me, and kissed my cheeks. Speaking a mile a minute, as if I understood (I didn't), she pulled me by the hand into the kitchen and motioned for me to pick a pasta, holding up over a dozen boxes for me to examine. I chose one that looked familiar: ziti.

At eight P.M., my friend's mother served the soup—the start of what was, for me, a very late dinner. While I spooned up mine more quickly than usual—I was starving—my hosts ate at a leisurely pace, the clank of their spoons punctuated with chatter, laughter, and hand waving. As the bowls were cleared and we began on the ziti, I made a conscious effort to slow my American pace.

They offered seconds on the ziti, and I accepted, to demonstrate my thanks for their hospitality. As I cleaned my plate, however, I realized too late that the ziti was only the second course. There were four more to come: a meat dish, a cheese plate, fruit, and a dessert. Although stuffed, I continued to eat. By the end of the meal, my eyes were bulging and my hosts, beaming.

I'm Italian by heritage and know meals in Italy can be lengthy affairs, but dazzled by the array of flavors, the joy at being reunited with my friend, and the celebratory nature of the meal, I'd accidentally overdone it. The social context of the meal had overwhelmed my personal awareness of hunger and fullness.

Whether we live in Perugia or Peoria, the unspoken rules that govern the behavior of a particular culture—called social norms—shape the way humans eat. Each day, in our corner of the planet, we face an endless array of social eating opportunities—snacks at work, wedding banquets, dinners or parties with friends. Because most of our eating is social in nature, we must be mindful of society's eating norms and of how a social environment affects our eating decisions.

More often than not, falling in line with these norms, which include the "new normal" of overeating, can make it tough to decide on healthy choices. A significant aspect of EI is being able to navigate relationships, which require that you communicate effectively, create strong boundaries, and respond rather than react to difficult social situations. These skills come into play when we eat with others. With a strong Eat.Q., you'll enjoy connecting with others without automatically—and sometimes unconsciously—adhering to these unhealthy eating "rules."

A Strong Eat.Q. Tunes You In to Eating Cues

If you want to know why you eat more while in others' company, here's one way to view the answer:

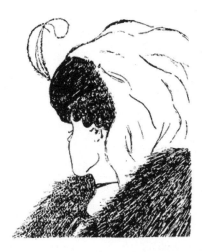

This illustration, with which you're probably familiar, is an example of what is called a *figure-ground illusion*. Look at the foreground, and you see an old woman. Focus on the background, and it's the face of a young woman in three-quarter view, wearing a feathered hat and fur coat. After you "see" both images, you can shift back and forth between them.

Like the illustration, social eating has a background and a foreground. The background is the external reality of the social event—the party, the wedding, your interactions with others. The foreground is your internal reality. When we eat with others, we typically focus on the background.

With a solid Eat.Q., you'll see both background and foreground, more easily shift back and forth between them, and be mindful of how the backdrop or context of the social event shapes your eating decisions.

I see social eating as driven by three main influences, which fall into either foreground or background.

Who's at the table (background)? Humans have a strong desire to be liked, and there is evidence that we mimic others to gain this acceptance and fit in.[1]

This behavioral mimicry is why we typically dress like our friends and use the same slang. It's also why we tend to eat like those around us, ordering similar foods, putting the same amount on our plates, and eating at the same pace. Whether the mimicking is intentional or unconscious (it can be either), your dining companions can significantly shape your food choices, research shows. Eat with people who order grilled-chicken salads, and you'll likely make healthier selections. Sit down with people who choose burgers and fries, and you're likely to follow suit.

If your eating and ordering style changes with your dining partners, you might be what I call an *eating chameleon*. Later in the chapter you'll learn to distinguish between people who help you eat well (I call them *helpers*) and those who hurt or even sabotage your efforts (*hinderers*).

Why are you at the table (background)? It can be a pleasure to eat, whether you're hungry or not. Yet in social situations, eating takes on a deeper significance. You eat to celebrate, share your love, bond with others. Without a strong Eat.Q., celebratory eating—weddings, holidays, anniversary parties, and the like—can get the better of you. As your Eat.Q. rises, you'll be able to share a meal without being swayed by others' choices. You'll also pick up on your partner's or the group's eating norms, whether spoken ("Let's order dessert!") or unspoken (*Everyone's ordering burgers*).

How do you feel when you're at the table (foreground)? You decide what to eat based on how you feel in the moment, and you're not always aware of those feelings. The EAT method can help you identify, embrace, and accept emotions, whatever they may be, and right there at the table, so you make better choices.

Your level of self-confidence or self-esteem can also drive your emotions. Can you recall the last time someone bullied you to eat, or eat more, when you weren't hungry, or you ate to the point of discomfort at a gathering of people you didn't know well because you felt anxious? Raising your Eat.Q. can help you find that balance between enjoying others' company and honoring your own needs and preferences. Let's look at each of these factors more closely.

QUIZ: ARE YOU A BACKGROUND EATER?

Eating with others has a *background* (the social context) and a *foreground* (your internal reality, which includes how you feel and how hungry or full you are). Some of us are more sensitive to background than others. The more you are swayed by social cues to eat, the more you will typically eat. This quiz measures your vulnerability to background eating.

1. When you eat, you would rather . . .

   a. eat alone, so you can have whatever you want in peace.

   b. eat alone, but turn on the TV for company.

   c. share a meal with one other person, a significant other or good friend.

   d. eat with a group of friends.

2. Your mother-in-law offers you a piece of her chocolate cake. You . . .

   a. politely decline, as many times as it takes. You honestly don't want any, thanks!

   b. accept a slice to be polite, but play with it on your plate.

   c. accept a slice, but request a very small piece. It's all you want, really.

   d. accept a slice whether you want it or not. If you didn't, you'd never hear the end of it.

3. You're having dinner with fit and health-conscious friends, who all order salads. You want a burger and fries. What do you order?

   a. The burger and fries.

   b. The burger, substituting a salad for the fries.

   c. A salad and a sandwich. Ham and cheese is healthier than a burger, right?

   d. Exactly what they order. You'd feel like a glutton eating "bad" food in front of them.

4. You're having lunch with your significant other, who eats at a breakneck speed. You . . .

   a. eat at your own pace. Your partner often ends up waiting for you to finish.

    b. eat slightly slower than your partner. Eating quickly upsets your stomach.

    c. notice yourself speeding up just a little.

    d. match your partner's pace, so you finish at the same time.

5. When you eat with others, you . . .

    a. eat as you please, whether you're at home or dining out.

    b. consider what your companions order, or how much they put on their plates, then follow suit.

    c. eat a bit less than normal, unless everyone's eating everything in sight.

    d. eat noticeably less than others. You tend to eat like a "good girl (or boy)" in front of others.

6. Your coworkers decide to hit the trendy new neighborhood bistro for dinner. You ate a late lunch. You . . .

    a. decline graciously. You just ate a few hours ago. Next time!

    b. go but order coffee. You just want to peek at the menu and check out the ambiance.

    c. go but eat lightly: soup and a salad.

    d. go and order a full dinner. Why not? It's an impromptu party!

SCORING

Give yourself zero points for each (a) answer, one point for each (b) answer, two points for each (c) answer, and three points for each (d) answer.

0–6 points: High Foreground, Low Background. While you can tune in to your hunger and satiety levels, you may skip social events to avoid overeating. As you raise your Eat.Q., you may find it easier to socialize at events that include eating.

7–12 points: Medium Foreground, High Background. You're aware that when you share a meal with others, it's easy for you to follow the crowd. As you raise your Eat.Q. and learn to honor your hunger and satiety, you'll be less likely to fall victim to groupthink (or, in this case, groupeat).

13–18 points: Low Foreground, High Background. If your group is overeating, so are you. If they're picking at salads, you are too, regardless of how hungry or full you feel. For you, to raise your Eat.Q. is to raise your self-awareness in general. No more being the last to order so you can copy what others do!

THE EAT METHOD MODEL OF SOCIAL EATING
When you eat with others, it's easy to fall into the when-in-Rome mind-set.

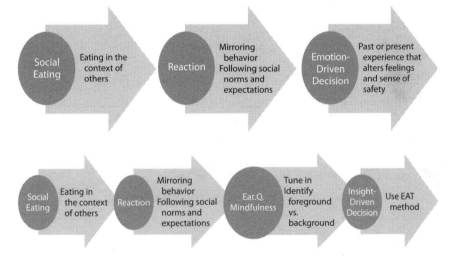

When you eat with others, it's easy to fall into the when-in-Rome mind-set. When you take a mindful pause and tune in to your foreground and background, it's easier to decide what and how much *you* want to eat, regardless of others' choices.

Who's at the Table: Helpers and Hinderers

Part of the E in the EAT method is to become aware of how other people influence your eating decisions, particularly in social situations. If you think about it, you'll usually be able to fit friends, family members, and coworkers into one of two categories.

Helpers have a healthy relationship with food. Their sensible eating habits and relaxed attitudes about what's on their plates—and yours—make it easier to eat well. The support they lavish on you may also help you lose weight. In a study of 267 overweight women, Stanford University researchers found that women who had frequent friend and family support were more likely to lose weight than those who didn't (72 percent versus 46 percent).[2]

Alas, *hinderers* seem to outnumber helpers. Either they judge or bully you about your choices, or "worry" that you'll waste away. As you read this section, try to identify the helpers and hinderers in your life, from your partner to your coworkers.

Helpers

I'm fortunate to have a helper in my life: my friend and colleague Susan (yes, another Susan!). I'm inspired by her calm, easy relationship with food. At fifty-five, she's at a healthy weight, and while eating is part of her world, it's not the center of it. She naturally helps those around her eat well; all you have to do is watch and copy.

Susan seems to be always in tune with her hunger. If she's invited to lunch and isn't hungry, she says "No thank you" with confidence and without apology. If she's up for socializing, she'll join us and order tea. No matter what others order, she never judges or comments; their choices are their business.

One day we ate lunch at a local restaurant. Afterward, the owner treated Susan to a lemon scone, a treat he knows Susan loves. Susan thanked him and said, "I'm so full, I'm going to take this home and enjoy it tonight!" Then she wrapped it in a napkin. Even when offered a favorite food—*on the house*—she considered her hunger level and made a wise decision.

If you have helpers like Susan in your life, model aspects of your eating decisions on theirs until they become second nature. If you don't have a helper, look for one. If you can't find one in your family or social circle, try an online support group.

The next best thing to finding a helper is to be one. When you eat with someone who you know struggles with food, consciously make healthy choices around him or her (perhaps at a wedding, party, or family dinner), and don't critique what's on that person's plate. When you act like a helper, you have the opportunity to practice EAT method principles and perhaps pass them along.

THE EAT.Q. KITCHEN

Cooking at home can significantly help you manage your weight, research has found. The good news is a variety of high- and low-tech kitchen gadgets can help even more, allowing you to break old unhealthy eating habits and make healthier food decisions easier.

The six kitchen tools below can help you tackle two of the most emotionally charged challenges you may encounter at your own kitchen table: eating slower and discerning healthy portion sizes. Both challenges are fraught with emotion—too much, too little, too fast, too slow, "It's so good I want *more*." These gadgets can assist you in navigating these challenges in smart and mindful ways.

1. **HAPIfork.** Eating too fast can cause you to eat much more than you planned. HAPIfork to the rescue! If you take more than one bite in ten seconds, this electronic fork vibrates and lights up, reminding you to slow down. The HAPIfork also measures how long it takes you to eat your meal, the amount of "fork servings" taken per minute, and the interval between fork servings. You can get apps for your PC and phone, too. See hapilabs.com/products-hapifork.asp. *Low-tech alternative:* Chopsticks slow you down, too, as long as you don't use them like a pro.

2. **Obol bowl.** Do you eat cereal too fast? If so, it's understandable. Healthy cereal dissolves quicker than junk food cereal due to the low sugar content. The Obol is divided into two sections—one for milk, one for cereal. The cereal portion slopes down to scoot the cereal into the milk, so you don't have to pour in your milk all at once. Voilà—eat at your own pace, mixing cereal with milk a little at a time, rather than worrying that your flakes will get soggy if you don't eat quick! See obol.co. *Low-tech alternative:* Pour your cereal in a regular bowl and your milk in a glass. Add a little milk at a time.

3. **Melon baller, cheese grater, apple wedger.** Research suggests that we're more likely to eat food presented in an aesthetically

pleasing way (this is why restaurants place a sprig of mint on a plate or drizzle balsamic vinaigrette around the edge of your entrée). If you already own these tools, start using them! You can add perfectly shaped melon balls to fruit salad, curly shavings of grated cheese to pasta, or a few pretty apple wedges next to your sandwich, making your meal look like it came out of a five-star kitchen. *Low-tech alternative*: Many garnishes are made with a simple paring knife. You can cut ribbons, flowers, and stars, for example, from vegetables like cucumbers and carrots.

4. **Bento boxes.** In Japanese, the word *bento* is derived from the word for "convenient" and this is what we're looking for in meals—easy and ready to go. More fun and green friendly than ordinary food containers, these attractive, simple boxes are common in Japanese homes for single-portion takeout or a home-packed meal. Keep them handy to box up leftovers immediately after you finish your evening meal so you're not tempted to eat extra portions or nibble on leftovers. See laptoplunches.com. *Low-tech alternative*: Serve yourself or your family lasagna, then immediately pop the rest into freezer bags—either individual or family-size portions. You can't nibble at it once it's frozen, and when you're ready to serve it again, simply leave it on the counter to defrost.

5. **Pasta measurer.** If you routinely toss a fistful of pasta into the pot, you often end up with far too much—and that extra can find its way onto your plate. This simple gadget looks like a ruler with holes from one to four portions. Simply slide the uncooked pasta through the appropriate hole, and you'll make just the right amount. *Low-tech alternative:* Use napkin ring holders of varying diameters. A holder with a ⅞-inch diameter equals one portion; a ring with a diameter of 1⅛ inches equals two portions. Use a 1½ -inch ring for three portions and a 1¾-inch ring for four portions.

Hinderers

Those who pressure you to eat, or shame and judge you when you do, can thwart your ability to develop a healthy relationship with food. While their behavior can be malicious, more often than not they feel they're being helpful. As we know, they aren't. Here are some of the things the hinderers in my clients' lives have said:

- "You look terrible! Your face is sagging. You're losing too fast."

- "It's your birthday. You can have a piece of cake."

- "You don't like my lasagna anymore?"

EXERCISE: TAKE THE EAT.Q. KITCHEN CHALLENGE

I challenge you for one week to:

1. Use at least two tools (high- or low-tech alternatives) to slow you down—the HAPIfork, chopsticks, bento boxes, etc.

2. Remove some electronics from your kitchen, or don't use them. While high-tech gadgets like food-tracking apps can help, they can also distract you if they're used in the kitchen, making it difficult to eat in a mindful way. If you have a TV in your kitchen, remove it; watching TV while you eat is one of the greatest prompters of overeating. Leave your mobile phone, laptop, remote control, and radio in the next room.

3. At least twice a day use one high- or low-tech tool that helps you slow down size instead of making an emotionally driven decision.

How did you like this challenge? Did you notice a change in your Eat.Q.? Use this self-awareness to help rearrange your kitchen—place the tools that were successful in slowing you down and guiding your portion sizes in a handy and easy-to-see location. I bet you will have a new appreciation for the tools in your kitchen!

NAME YOUR EATING HELPERS AND HINDERERS

I often ask my clients to identify the people in their lives who support or sabotage their efforts to eat well. I invite you to consider the same question. This simple but powerful exercise can help you embrace and accept the helpful or hurtful influence of family, friends, and others on your eating.

1. Think of the people you see regularly: your partner, children, friends, coworkers, and so on. Even if you see them only on holidays or at other special times, include them on your list.

2. Add a line or two about how each person on your list encourages or attempts to derail your efforts to eat well. (If you have more hinderers than helpers, join the crowd. Most of my clients do too.)

My Helpers

1. _____

2. _____

3. _____

4. _____

5. _____

My Hinderers

1. _____

2. _____

3. _____

4. _____

5. _____

- "There's one doughnut left. Want it?"

- "You're no fun since you started this diet."

One of my clients, Holly, had two hinderers in her life: her mother and her husband. As a child, if Holly ate french fries, her mother traced her finger in the air, up and down Holly's figure, as a silent rebuke. A day later, she'd take Holly out for ice cream, "just the two of us." The conflicting messages continued into adulthood. At family dinners, if Holly had a second helping of mashed potatoes, her mother would raise an eyebrow but heckle her if she didn't eat a slice of her homemade pie for dessert.

Her husband's preferred tactic was sabotage. Holly would shop on Sunday and plan a stellar healthy meal. Coincidentally, Monday night her husband wanted pizza. The grilled chicken and roasted veggies meal would be wrapped up, and Holly would eat too much pizza.

I focused on helping Holly raise her awareness of the feelings her hinderers aroused in her: shame, helplessness, and anger. Once aware of them, she could learn to press PAUSE when she identified them, manage them, and make an insight-driven decision. Here's Holly's EAT method "prescription":

E: While the comments Holly's hinderers made always hurt, they'd become so ingrained that she almost didn't hear them anymore. I asked her to carry a tiny notebook and list each and every comment as it was made—what it was, who made it, the situation, and how it made her feel. Once she began her log, she was surprised to discover how often these comments popped up.

A: I had Holly use her log to connect her eating behavior with the feelings the comments aroused in her. She found that the comments usually propelled her into negative thinking: *Well, she thinks I'm fat, so I'll just* be *fat* or *He wants pizza? Fine. He'll just have to deal with my fat bum.* In most cases, Holly wasn't aware of the anger and negativity that triggered her self-sabotaging behavior.

T: When hinderers are truly hurtful, limiting contact may be the only option. Holly chose to spend less time with her mother, whose criticism wasn't limited to her daughter's food selections. She also began to eat before her husband arrived home from work, a sensible portion of healthy food she liked. Holly found one tool—Mental Makeover: Reframe That Feeling (tool 10 on page 249)—particularly helpful. It taught her to engage in positive self-talk to counteract the effect of her hinderers' comments on her feelings and decisions.

Before long, Holly's stronger inner voice drowned out their hurtful comments. These days, more often than not, she sticks to her healthy eating plan.

SET YOUR BOUNDARIES!

If you have a hinderer in your life, it's essential to become aware of and hold your boundaries. A boundary is a limit that separates you from others. Boundaries empower us to choose how we want to be treated by others. Boundaries also protect us. Whether you're talking about food or relationships, boundaries are helpful and necessary to prevent us from getting emotionally trampled or isolated from others. People with strong EI know how to set boundaries and maintain them effectively.

Setting boundaries doesn't require you to be rude. It just requires you to tune in to where your boundaries are and the points at which you feel they're being pushed or violated. Here are two ways to set boundaries:

First, practice your "no." One reason the word no may be hard to say is because it sounds so foreign to our own ears! That's why it's helpful to literally practice turning down food you don't want. If you find it helpful, practice in front of a mirror until your refusal sounds effortless and confident. The no should be clear but kind, the tone light but firm. You can use the following examples or come up with your own.

- "No, thank you. I don't want to share a dessert."

- "It looks delicious, but really, no thanks."

- "I'm fine right now. I'll take a piece for later."

Who's at the Table: Eating to Blend In

The tree-dwelling lizards called chameleons have two unique abilities. They can move each eye independently of the other, and they can change color. The latter change isn't triggered by the color of the chameleon's surroundings, as is commonly thought, but by light, temperature, and nervous stimulation, such as anger or fear. Even so, this unique ability to match its surroundings makes me think of another way humans tend to act when they eat with others: they try to blend in.

To some extent we're all chameleons, whether we're conscious of it or

- "It's tough to refuse such a wonderful cook, but I'm stuffed, thanks."

Second, use a variety of boundaries. Besides verbal boundaries like the ones above, there are two other types you can use.

Physical boundaries are about adding literal space and distance between your body or things, or putting limits on how and when things can be touched:

- "This is my snack drawer, and that drawer is yours (or your side of the refrigerator)."
- "Please keep your snacks somewhere I can't see them. Thank you."

Time boundaries are specific limits on how long you engage in an activity rather than an undefined or unlimited amount of time:

- "I can stay five minutes, and then I have to leave."
- "I'm sorry, but I really can't stay. I have an appointment in twenty minutes."

It's important to be aware that your hinderer may test your boundaries, so be ready to stand your ground. With patience and repetition, you'll find it easier to say no and stick to your guns!

not. Behavioral mimicry dictates that if you eat with someone who tends to eat more than you do, you're likely to eat more, and vice versa.

Charlotte was a classic chameleon eater. At around the same time that her suits started to feel snug, this smart, hard-driving advertising executive landed the account of an upscale line of natural foods. Frustrated, she called me for help. Her job was her life, this account was important to her, and she *would* lose the weight.

I quizzed her extensively on what I call the W questions: *What* was she eating, *when, where, with whom,* and *why?*

Based on her answers, and the food diary she kept for a week, Charlotte had no issues with the usual suspects, such as low nutrition knowledge or no access to healthy food. What struck me was her inconsistent eating pattern.

HOW YOU EAT, ALL BY YOURSELF

When I opened the sweet and quirky book *What We Eat When We Eat Alone,*[4] I was, ironically, alone on a train riding from Philadelphia to New York City. I'd just finished a dinner I'd packed myself, which featured my very favorite foods: Greek yogurt, cheddar cheese and soy crisps, and chicken salad—a weird conglomeration. I was going for a mix of mindful convenience, but my meal involved a measure of both pleasure and comfort. My sister, who knows I love chicken salad, had made it just for me to enjoy on my journey.

What We Eat When We Eat Alone served as a good launching point for me to think about how we eat when no one's around versus when we're in a social realm, and why. I invite you to ponder this for just a moment. Do you, in your anonymity, break convention—eat with your fingers or indulge food quirks? (A friend of a friend, a woman nearing seventy, still crumbles cookies into her vegetable soup, a habit acquired during her first pregnancy.) In a restaurant, do you order a dish that would surprise or even shock those who know you (a vegetarian enjoying a veal chop!)? At home, do you cook a ready-made pizza that you buy for your children but secretly covet?

In a single day, she could eat a stir-fry and a steak sandwich, a grilled-chicken salad and chicken wings. The amount she ate also varied wildly: some meals were characterized by sensible portions, while others seemed more like binges. (Bingers often feel out of control.) What was going on?

As it turned out, nothing I hadn't seen before: chameleon eating. On the job, her colleagues ate sushi or salad, with dressing on the side, as they talked business in the boardroom, so Charlotte did too. At home, her husband ate pizza, fried chicken, and burgers, so Charlotte followed suit. (Several studies have documented such unhealthy "copycat eating" in couples.)[3]

In a perfect world, your friends, coworkers, and family members would eat well, and you'd sit next to them and mimic their healthy food choices. As it is, you need to use your Eat.Q.

Just as important: how much do you eat? Research suggests that we eat less when we're alone, but my client base includes a fair number of people who eat healthy in front of others—grilled chicken, soup and salad, a bun-less burger and a side of veggies—only to let loose when they're alone.

How about you? Is there a public you, who eats modest portions of healthy food when you're around others, and a private you, who lets loose with food when you're alone?

Ponder this, too: Is there a distinction between your solo and your social eating? If you typically eat radically differently when you're alone, could it be that you feel embarrassed? Are you unwilling to let others see you engage in what you consider a very private activity?

Answering such questions is the first step to raising your Eat.Q. The second is practicing a mindful pause to gain access to and manage any self-defeating patterns you may find. Finally, you can turn to tools that help you manage those feelings and make wise eating decisions.

ME VERSUS WE

Kate came to see me nine months after she'd gotten married. Struggling with posthoneymoon weight gain, the twenty-nine-year-old teacher placed the blame squarely on her new husband, Brad.

"Before I met him, I ate mostly vegetarian," Kate told me. "But Brad's always been a meat-and-potatoes guy, and without me realizing it, I started to eat what he ate—BBQ-pulled-pork sandwiches, huge burgers, ice cream after dinner." Kate was considering adopting a vegetarian lifestyle again but worried they would drift apart—meals were the only times they actually slowed down and talked. Would they lose that precious "couple time" and begin to eat separately?

Kate had fallen into a trap I call Eating Under the Influence of Love. In this phenomenon, one or both partners gain or lose weight (usually gain) when they enter a new relationship. In fact, research shows that couples display a convergence of eating behaviors—that is, they tend to eat the same foods and gain and lose similar amounts of weight.[5]

That's no surprise—eating together is an early part of the courtship process (sharing popcorn at the movies, snuggling up at home with a pizza and Netflix, going out for ice cream). Eating isn't just a pleasurable activity; it's a bonding one.

Later, as couples become more entwined in each other's lives, they share similar routines and patterns—they eat at the same time of day and shop for groceries together. Individual eating styles fade away; it's simply easier to prepare one meal than two.

My work with Kate focused on helping her shift from trying to change Brad's eating to finding ways they could mesh their eating styles. Here are a few tips I gave her and give to other couples as well; they can work for you, too.

1. Relinquish control. At first, Kate tried to revamp Brad's menu, serving him tofu and grilled vegetable salads. It didn't work. Trying to change the way your significant other eats is a battle you can't win; it only results in a battle for control. Accept

that, for better or worse, you are each in charge of your own plate.

2. Be a good role model. *Show,* don't *tell,* your healthy choices. In other words, don't tell your partner you're ordering fish instead of ribs. Just do it. I assured Kate that, over time, Brad might begin eating healthier on his own because we are susceptible to mimicking the behavior of others.

3. Reinforce your partner's healthy choices. If you're lucky, your partner wants to improve his eating habits. But support is found in reinforcement, not control. For example, you might say, "Great choice!" when he chooses the salad over the fries or buy low-fat ice cream rather than the full-fat gourmet ice cream he (and you!) can't resist.

4. Compromise. Take turns buying your favorite foods. If you like low-fat yogurt and your significant other doesn't, find a percent somewhere in between.

5. Challenge each other. Healthy competition can ignite the spark between a couple. Rather than set up a weight-loss challenge, find ways to compete around adding healthy behaviors to your eating. Who can find the yummiest recipes that are also healthy, make the hottest homemade salsa, whip up the tastiest marinade for your grilled chicken, or grill vegetables to perfection?

6. Layer your meals. If you cook together, create a "base" meal—pasta, pizza, salads—and layer on ingredients specific to your particular tastes. Kate and Brad often ate salads for dinner, a perfect base meal. He'd top his with steak, blue cheese dressing, and croutons. She'd add balsamic vinaigrette, grilled vegetables, and a few shavings of fresh Parmesan cheese.

As Kate learned, it's possible to be in a relationship and honor your own feelings, and then make choices based on those feelings.

Why You're at the Table

Years ago, when I lived in Japan, my friend introduced me to virtually everyone in her community. (I felt a bit like a celebrity.) At each stop, as is the Japanese custom, my host offered me something to eat or drink. At one stop, however, my host offered me a cup of something clear and jiggly. Its consistency made my stomach turn; to me, it looked like, well, mucus. *Ugh.*

I must have made a face, because my friend leaned forward and whispered urgently, "You *must* eat it."

I knew that. My host would have perceived my refusal as an insult and a disgrace. At that moment, the background—the symbolic importance

WOMEN AND COPYCAT NOSHING

Lunch with a girlfriend. The girls' night out. Women sharing meals can forge new friendships or strengthen established ones. But women who eat together tend to match each other bite for bite, a recent Dutch study suggests.[6]

Researchers call this *behavioral mimicry:* the process in which one person unknowingly imitates another's behavior. Mimicry may be related to the neural link between perception and action. That is, perceiving another person's movements activates *your* motor system for that same movement, which in turn increases your likelihood of initiating the same movement.

In this study, researchers took a look at the eating patterns of seventy pairs of women as they dined together in a lab arranged to resemble a bar. Each pair was served a full meal that they had twenty minutes to eat. One woman in each pair knew in advance how much food she would be served, but neither was told how much to eat.

The researchers catalogued the timing of each bite—3,888 bites in all—to determine how many bites were the product of mimicry. The scientists distinguished between mimicked bites (those taken within five seconds of the other person taking a bite) and non-mimicked bites (those taken outside the five-second interval).

behind eating this unappetizing dish—outweighed my foreground. So, I put on my game face and choked it down. (You know, it wasn't bad—just mild-flavored bean-curd paste).

When you eat with other people, you must constantly negotiate your foreground and background. That is, you must balance what the food means to *you*—and how well it meets your hunger, needs, tastes, and preferences—with what your acceptance of it means to *others* (care, intimacy, respect, politeness). Here are some examples:

- cooking for someone who is sick, or bringing over a homemade dish after a funeral, to show you care

After analyzing each bite, the researchers determined that both women in the pairs were quite likely to take a forkful of food at the same time. While each woman in the pairs mimicked the other, the partner who knew her portion size in advance was less likely to mimic her companion.

The researchers also found that women were three times as likely to mimic their dining companion during the first ten minutes of the meal as in the last ten minutes. The researchers suspect this is because the beginning of a meal is when a person begins to establish rapport with a stranger.

Why the mimicry? The researchers raised two possibilities. Both women may be unconsciously primed to mimic each other by what is called a "mirroring network." In this case, one of the women sees the other lift her fork and take a bite, so she automatically does the same. The other possibility is that the women were monitoring each other to avoid eating "inappropriately" or to ingratiate themselves with their eating companions. Researchers also speculated that mimicry may lessen when eating with familiar people compared to strangers.

The next time you're sharing a meal, do a quick "background check" (yes, right at the table). Are you raising and lowering your fork in rhythm with hers? If so, you know what to do.

- cooking a romantic meal to create a sense of intimacy

- preparing the holiday meal that grandmother used to make to bond the family

- taking part in celebrations that focus on ritual (a seder meal in the Jewish culture, for example) or family (holidays, a wedding or post-funeral buffet, and the like)

These examples highlight some of the best things in life: good food and good family and friends to share it with. That's why holiday eating is so problematic. Every year from Christmas to New Year's Day, and again during the spring holidays, my clients must shift back and forth between background and foreground, between displaying graciousness and love to their hosts and honoring themselves. Indeed, we all do this dance, some of us more successfully than others.

If you're at the table because you're partaking in a meal with a symbolic meaning, using your Eat.Q. can help you balance this deep—at times, primal—pull to eat with your desire to eat healthy food in sensible portions.

Once you raise your Eat.Q., you'll treat these special meals the same way you do everyday meals. The background of the social event won't give you a license or excuse to overeat. You'll focus on the foreground—your internal reality. You'll pick and choose what is truly special and unique to the meal—maybe a food you get once a year—and enjoy an amount that satisfies both your physical hunger and your desire for connection and pleasure.

How We Feel When We're at the Table

Social gatherings can inflame emotions to especially high levels. The following are some feelings that commonly lead to overeating in social situations.

A Desire to Please

How many times have you eaten an extra helping or accepted dessert because you wanted to make someone happy? People with a strong desire to please others tend to overeat in social situations, even if they're not hungry, a study published in the *Journal of Social and Clinical Psychology* found.

They're also more likely to indulge in foods they'd normally avoid, such as fatty snacks and desserts.[7] If you enter a social gathering aware that you like to please others, you'll stand a better chance of following your hunger rather than the crowd. Don't give yourself the opportunity to cave in to other people's expectations. Order or choose your food first to avoid people-pleasing.

Anger

Five minutes before you sit down with your family to Christmas dinner, you had to endure your sister-in-law's boasting about her new home, angelic kids,

---

WE BITES AND ME BITES

In the following exercise, your task is to turn on your full awareness to alter unconscious mirroring behavior.

1. Choose someone you eat with frequently—a partner, coworker, or friend.

2. Before you meet up with your dining companion, decide how hungry you are, so you won't be influenced by what he or she orders. Are you ravenous? Slightly hungry?

3. As you begin your meal or snack with your companion, make a conscious effort to step out of sync with him or her. Take a deep breath. Focus inward. Assess your level of hunger from one to ten. Focus your attention. Before you take a bite, ask yourself if this a "we" bite or a "me" bite. In other words, are you taking this particular bite in tandem with your companion, or does it reflect your own sense of hunger or fullness? Occasionally, set limits for yourself, either in your head or stated aloud to your companion, such as "You're still eating but I'm done. I'll sit here and chat with you."

4. After you say good-bye, check in with yourself. Did you eat less, more, or about the same as usual with this comparison?

and big promotion. You're boiling with irritation, anger, maybe even rage. However, eating more than you know you should isn't the answer.

Somehow, taking out anger on yourself seems more acceptable than expressing it to others. (As the twelve-step program expression goes, "I'll show you, I'll hurt me.") To reduce anger-driven overeating, however, you need to cope with anger directly. If you must attend a gathering where you know you'll feel anger—say, a family reunion or holiday dinner—arm yourself with a few strategies to cope with your anger in safe and productive ways. For example, to help lighten your mood, look for the irony in or the humorous side of the situation. For extra help, use tools 13 and 15 (pages 254 and 259).

Loneliness

You can have a spouse and a circle of friends and still feel a profound sense of loneliness from time to time. If you view food as a substitute for connection and companionship, perhaps it's because in your experience food chases away loneliness. In fact, a study conducted at the University at Buffalo, SUNY, suggests that the emotional power of comfort food (such as chicken soup) comes from its connection with relationships.[8] In other words, through comfort food, you *can* "go home again."

Or try to, at least. It's not the food itself that drives away loneliness. It's the emotions it evokes. While getting that distinction isn't always easy, the EAT method can help you break away from illusory comfort and choose comfort that's real.

Trying to ease the void of loneliness with food can actually widen the chasm you perceive between yourself and others. If you feel ashamed or uncomfortable in your body, you may react by retreating from the world. Only genuine connection can ease loneliness. It can be helpful to first accept that you're feeling isolated, and writing can help you come to terms with the desire to connect. If loneliness prompts you to overeat, try the writing exercise in tool 15 (page 259).

Joy

At many social events, eating and happiness go hand in hand—weddings, birthdays, a promotion at work. When you feel good, you want the feelings to stay. It's easy to keep eating to hold on to those positive feelings just a bit longer. A piece of cake tastes so good and you don't want to let go of the moment of joy it gives you, so you eat another.

It's okay to experience joy when you eat. But perhaps in school or university economics class you learned about the law of diminishing returns, which states that as more investment is made, overall return on that investment increases at a declining rate. Eating is governed by a similar principle. At first, more food intensifies joy. But after a certain point, more food doesn't result in more joy. In fact, as you cross from enjoying a good meal into overeating, that joy can turn to pain. Savoring your food—eating mindfully—can help you gain the sensory joy of eating without going overboard. See tool 7 for instructions (page 240).

Competition

Some of my clients are surprised to find that eating with others brings out their competitive streak. Sometimes, women compete to be the one in their group who eats the least or orders the meal with the least number of calories. Men have also told me stories about how they vied to be the guy who eats the *most*—who devours the most wings or finishes the biggest steak. While competitiveness in social eating doesn't always fall so neatly along gender lines, such feelings can influence what you order and how much you eat.

If eating with another person, or a group, brings out the competitor in you, examine your motivations closely. Ask yourself what you win by eating the least, or most. A sense of control or mastery perhaps? If so, why do you seek it? Will acting on such competitive feelings while eating with others foster intimacy or thwart it? Remember to focus on your own needs. Use the self-awareness exercises in this book to help you understand why you're driven to compete.

The Eat.Q. Solution: Celebrating People, Not Food

Even if you know that social eating is a challenge for you, please don't avoid it. Missing a family event or an office outing is a surefire way to arouse self-defeating emotions, such as guilt, anger, and loneliness, and you'll have missed an opportunity to practice the new skills you're learning.

So go. But before you leave the house, practice your mindful pause and review the tools you'll turn to if you feel a snap decision or a what-the-hell moment coming on. When you arrive at the event, switch back and forth between background and foreground to keep your awareness high.

Here's the core of the EAT method for social eating:

E: Observe Your Background

If you find it hard to manage your eating, the adage "When in Rome, do as the Romans do" does not always serve you well. In EAT method strategy, the expression is more like "When in Rome, observe the Romans first." To observe your background, pay attention to

- the seating arrangements. Is there assigned seating, or do you choose who you sit next to? (Sit next to a helper, if possible.)

- what the seating arrangements may tell you about the power dynamics of the table. Who sits at the head of the table? Who orders first?

- how the food is served. Is it buffet-style, where you serve yourself? Does the host make up and pass you your plate? Or are you given proportioned servings of food, as at a wedding banquet?

- the portion sizes of your dining companions or the crowd. Who is eating what you deem to be a moderate amount of food? Who seems to be overindulging? Are most people taking seconds or even thirds?

- the mood of the event. Is it raucous, like a party, or dignified, like a business dinner or cocktail party?

- how quickly or slowly your companions are eating.

- whether they are eating the same foods or ordering different foods.

- whether your judgments about a particular person are influencing your eating. For example, *I want to be thin like her* or *I'm not ordering that because I don't want to be his size.*

Attune yourself with the nuances, customs, and unspoken rules that may not be obvious at first glance. Then, consciously decide if it's wise to follow suit. If you observe others and check your foreground, you won't do as the Romans do and regret it.

A: Tune In to Your Foreground

Connect the dots between what's going on in the room and what's going on with you. Here are several ways to do it:

- Focus on your *hunger*. Let's say your spouse falls into his or her chair at a restaurant and announces, "I'm starved! Let's get an appetizer. In fact, let's both get one so we can share." Size up your hunger. Investigate it closely. Are you very hungry or just a little hungry? Decide which it is and order accordingly. On autopilot, you might fall into line without a second thought. But having sized up your hunger, you decide against it. You've consciously made the contrast between yourself and others very apparent.

- Focus on your *emotions*. Let's say you are silently fuming and feel manipulated into having dinner with your boss. You could order a string of rich, pricey dishes because he's picking up the tab, or you could manage your annoyance and select a healthy, sensible entrée that you know you'll enjoy.

- Focus on the *symbolism* of the meal. As we've just seen, food is imbued with relational meaning, which may lead you to unconsciously eat more to acknowledge the significance of a meal. A meal cooked for you by your mother is an expression of nurturing. An anniversary dinner implies connection and romance. Typically, however, a meal at the drive-through has no meaning other than it's after six P.M. and time to eat. Take a moment before you eat with others to examine whether this meal holds a deeper symbolic meaning. If so, ask yourself how this affects your decisions.

T: Turn to People Rather than Food

In our food-centric culture, it's sometimes hard to remember that, at its most primal level, sharing a meal is about connecting with others—reaffirming family bonds (holiday dinners), honoring rites of passage (weddings, graduations, birthday parties), or being a gracious host and enjoying each other's company, as my friend and her mother in Perugia illustrated so well.

Whatever the social situation, food is the means, not the end. Make it a point to talk to those around you rather than turning to food. Ask them questions. Really listen. The best way to manage social eating is to focus more on the social and less on the eating.

Your Plate Portion Portfolio

On Wall Street, successful investors balance taking risks and playing it safe. The former can lead to big payoffs—or losing everything. And yet, avoiding risk entirely can lead to stagnation and lack of growth. To manage risk, investors create a diversified portfolio of stocks and bonds—some that are high yield but risky, some that are low yield but safe, and some that are neither too risky nor too safe.

My financial wizard friend, John, advises his clients to diversify and helps them manage their strong desire for short-term profit and focus on long-term gains. And it got me to thinking: the advice that works for John's clients works with eating, too. Instead of managing risk with stocks and bonds, you're managing the *risky nature of impulses* with the foods you choose to put on your plate. I call it the plate portion portfolio, and it helps you find that balance between holding your ground and taking a leap. Notice that it isn't about restricting what you eat. Instead, it's about coping with your impulses.

High yield, high risk: Desserts, sweets, comfort foods, and holiday favorites. These foods tug at your impulses. They promise immediate gratification. They give you a lot of payoff quickly (they taste great!) but can lead to high losses (guilt, feeling overly full).

Low yield, low risk: Grilled chicken, salads, fruits, egg-white omelets, and other low-calorie but nutrient-dense foods. These foods generally don't lead to impulsive eating. They may not give you the immediate payoff (the high-intensity zing your taste buds crave) but they prevent you from overeating.

Moderate yield, moderate risk: Baked potatoes, chili, breads, and pasta salad. Sometimes these are foods that you want now. Generally, however, I consider them foods that don't press as heavily on your urges and cravings.

Five Steps to a Diversified Plate

At social events—from cocktail parties to Christmas dinner, with countless weddings, dinner parties, cookouts, and brunches in between—it's tempting to go heavy on the treats and skip the healthy options. With the perfectly portioned plate portfolio, you evenly distribute low-, medium-, and high-risk foods on your plate. This strategy can help you diversify your options, raising the odds that you don't overeat due to your impulses, as it helps ensure that you partake in some of the foods you love without eating too much of them.

When you attend a social event that involves food, mentally divide your plate like the graphic below. You can divide your plate any way you like—thirds, quarters, even halves. The point is to diversify your food choices.

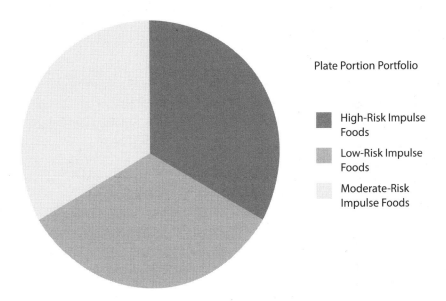

Plate Portion Portfolio

High-Risk Impulse Foods

Low-Risk Impulse Foods

Moderate-Risk Impulse Foods

1. Put the low-risk foods on your plate so you don't run out of room. If you want to play it safe, make the healthy foods section slightly bigger.

2. Add the moderate-risk foods.

3. Add the high-risk foods—one layer only, and only those that you like best.

4. Before you take a bite, look at your plate and give it a once-over. Ask yourself, what are the potential downsides of eating this five minutes after you finish it? It's a good way to weigh the short- and long-term gains of eating this food.

5. Double-check your impulses. If you had to take just one thing off your plate, what would it be? Sometimes you think you want a particular food but after a moment of reflection, you realize it is like an impulse buy that you'd regret later.

The Last Bite

"A party without a cake is just a meeting." This witty quote by Julia Child says what we all know to be true: food is an essential part of many celebrations. And yet, food is not the *only* part. Whether you're attending a baby shower, holiday feast, dinner date, or birthday party, you use your Eat.Q. to make a conscious choice about what and how much *you* want to eat, rather than letting others dictate your plate. You'll know you're on the right track when you can experience the food as one aspect of the social experience rather than as the focal point. If you tune in to your hunger and how you feel in the moment—anxious? giddy? lonely?—you'll learn how to truly enjoy food.

7

Stress

I work near a small city in Ohio that is home to large German and Amish communities. As I walk down Main Street, I sometimes hear people conversing in German. And in my office, sitting across from a stressed-out young woman—a recent arrival from Germany—was where I first heard the word *kummerspeck.*

Just a year in the United States, she had moved due to her husband's job transfer. I expected that she would have transitional issues related to loneliness, acclimating to a new country, and leaving friends and family behind.

food for THOUGHT

- When you're under emotional or physical stress, how do your decisions around food change?
- When you feel overwhelmed, what thoughts run through your mind? What do you tell yourself?
- Describe how emotional stress feels in your body. Does it manifest as a headache, a nervous stomach, fatigue?
- When you're under stress, do you tend to make snap decisions or deliberate endlessly, including about what to eat?
- What potential coping mechanisms besides eating do you have?

However, on her paperwork, Hilga had listed self-esteem and weight loss as her main goals for therapy. But soon after we started her first session, she said she already knew what her problem was.

"I have *kummerspeck*," she said.

I'd never heard *this* on Main Street, and I asked her what it was. She fumbled for words. "This is the weight you gain when you are worried about something," she said.

I was amazed: Germans have a word to describe stress eating. After she left, I looked up the word. Its literal translation is "grief bacon."

We all experience stress to some degree, and it isn't always negative. There's a world of difference between *eustress*—the positive, butterflies-in-the-stomach excitement you experience when you land a promotion or prepare for a new baby—and *distress*—the anxiety that gives you headaches and insomnia.

There's also a difference between acute and chronic stress. Acute stress is temporary, such as you experience when caught in a traffic jam. Chronic stress grinds on endlessly—perhaps due to a strained relationship, occupational burnout, ongoing financial worries—and is the kind of stress associated with increased risk of heart disease and other chronic diseases. Either kind can lead you to what we know as stress eating.

Strictly speaking, stress is not an emotion. It's a symptom of negative feelings, such as anxiety or anger—feelings that stem from your perception of the stressor rather than the stressor itself. Left unchecked, chronic stress can do more than deplete your zest for life. It can actually increase belly fat, and it's associated with health problems such as type 2 diabetes and heart disease, an outcome that leads to even more stress.[1]

The bad news is that people who have a strong EI actually are more tuned in to when they are stressed out—in other words, they are more aware of being stressed. The good news, however, is that they often have better emotional resources for coping with that stress, such as self-talk, social support, and relaxation. While you can't wave a magic wand and make stress disappear, you can learn to manage it and reduce its negative impact on your life and waistline. In this chapter, you'll learn to identify your unique response to stress and perceive, predict, and prepare for stress's impact on your eating. Both skills will help you break a pattern of emotion-driven eating triggered primarily by stress.

This Is Your Life on Stress

One day I was visiting a friend who has a toddler son and a daughter in nursery. As we chatted in the kitchen, the little girl colored a picture, working hard to stay within the lines. All was peaceful until, suddenly, her brother snatched her picture and tore it in two. I braced myself for a meltdown. Instead, the little girl rose silently from the table, sat on the floor, and assumed what appeared to be the lotus position.

"What are you doing?" I asked, surprised and amused.

Eyes closed, she replied, "My teacher taught us to do this when we're mad."

I don't know about you, but I was never taught how to deal with stress or anger at any point in my formal education, let alone nursery. I was impressed. Perhaps this little girl was already learning that you don't need food to soothe negative feelings; there are other, more positive ways to chill out.

Many of us aren't as fortunate. The American Psychological Association's 2012 report *Stress in America: Our Health at Risk* found that stress had risen in the past year for 39 percent of their respondents. Those who suffered from depression or who were overweight reported significantly higher average stress levels than the rest of the population and were much more likely to say they didn't think they were doing enough to manage their stress.[2] According to a study by the Mental Health Foundation, 59 percent of respondents in the UK indicated that over the last five years they had felt stressed. In 2012 the Australian Psychological Society conducted a survey of 1552 people over the age of 18. Nearly a quarter of respondents reported suffering from moderate to severe levels of stress. Behind these findings are real people, perilously close to burnout—and it's likely that many of them use food to cool the heat of stress.

All the more reason to boost your EI skills. Emotional intelligence and the ability to manage stress go hand in hand. High-EI people can change their perception of a stressor to ramp down their physiological and psychological responses. They can talk themselves down with thoughts like *I can handle this* or *It's no big deal,* call a friend to vent, and generally let go. (More on letting go in a few pages.) By contrast, people with few EI skills struggle against the stressor, brooding and obsessing until they're emotionally and physically depleted. Worse, they may not be able to identify or verbalize their stress at all (chapter 3). Negative self-talk, in particular, makes stress feel more overwhelming and can trigger fight-or-flight responses.

Even with their backs against the wall, many people try to wait out the stress that diminishes their lives and widens their waistlines. Indeed, many of my clients tell me they'll tackle their eating when their relationship smoothes out, the divorce is final, or the deadline at work is past. But stress is a constant; while it waxes and wanes, it's never completely absent. This entails using your emotional intelligence to become an expert on how you experience stress—how it manifests in you, and how it affects your cravings, appetite, and eating decisions.

The first step is to perceive that stress is happening to you, and it affects your body, your brain, and the way you think, feel, and behave. This may sound obvious, but when you live at warp speed, as many of my clients do—frantically juggling jobs, kids, errands, meetings, classes—there isn't time to grasp the obvious. The obvious is thrust upon you after weeks of sleepless nights, months of irritability or emotional outbursts, or the sudden realization—*When did this happen?*—that nothing in your closet fits.

What's the solution? You heard it mentioned back in chapter 2: perceive, predict, prepare. I call this strategy *Triple P.* In practice it's the grown-up version of the little girl's response to her brother's behavior. But first, let's get to the ground zero of the stress–overeating connection: an automatic, primitive response to stress that alters our bodies and brains, thoughts and behavior.

Fight-or-Flight and the Big-Belly Plight

To understand why you feel you *must* eat that cupcake the moment stress hits, it's essential to learn the fundamentals of stress biology. It's complex, but here's what you need to know.

More than seventy-five years ago endocrinologist Hans Selye, recognizing the link between stress and illness, broke the stress response into three stages.[3]

In the *alarm stage,* which occurs when you're scared or under threat, your body enters fight-or-flight mode. Hardwired into your brain to help you identify a threat to your survival, the fight-or-flight response is your body's home alarm system. The area of the brain that controls the release of cortisol is called the HPA (hypothalamic-pituitary-adrenal axis). The instant it identifies danger, your body's sympathetic nervous system releases stress hormones, such as adrenaline and cortisol. These hormones take your body to a state of hyperarousal, so you're ready to fight the threat or run away.

When the body is in fight-or-flight mode, its key systems are amped up. Breathing quickens, which helps disperse more oxygen throughout the body. The heart beats faster, which increases the flow of blood to carry more oxygen to muscles. Blood sugar increases, so your body has the fuel it needs to fight or run. This is the kind of hyperarousal that allows a mother to lift a car to save her child.

After the immediate threat has passed, in the *resistance stage* your body tries to adapt to the continued stress. If the stress passes, you can start to rebuild your defenses.

In the short term, fight-or-flight responses can save your life. But if the stress never shuts off—if stress hormones *stay* elevated—your body moves into the *exhaustion stage*. Continued stress depletes your body, suppressing your immune defenses and increasing your risk for disease.[4]

In our caveman ancestors, fight-or-flight mode was tripped only in life-or-death situations, such as an encounter with a predator, and it powered down when the threat passed. Today, screaming kids, a ringing phone, or a full inbox can set off that primitive, powerful, automatic response designed to save your life.

The stress–weight gain connection centers on cortisol, which mobilizes the body's storage of fat and sugar to fight or flee and directs you to search for calorie-dense foods—specifically, foods stuffed with dietary fat and sugar.[5] Previous studies have found clear associations between altered stress responses and obesity.[6]

Stress can inflate your middle, too. Research associates depression, anxiety, and tension—all markers of stress—with the accumulation of visceral fat. While you tend to eat more when you're stressed, what you eat is also a factor. Typically, people under stress reach for what we call comfort foods and what researchers call reward foods: anything salty, sweet, or creamy. Another significant factor is the stress hormone response. Cortisol in particular seems to influence fat accumulation around the abdominal area.[7]

Higher-than-normal cortisol levels have been linked to weight gain even in the *absence* of a stressful event. In a small University of Michigan study, researchers boosted cortisol levels in people by directly stimulating their pituitary glands (no stress-inducing tasks involved) to see if it affected their eating behavior. It did; the participants ate more high-fat, sweet, and salty snacks. In essence, if a higher-than-normal amount of cortisol is pumping through your body, you're likely to be experiencing cravings.[8] No wonder it feels so difficult to say no to comfort foods!

Humans need energy—calories—to fight danger or flee it. From your body's point of view, turning to high-fat, calorie-dense foods, such as ice cream and chocolate, is a reasonable response to the all-consuming "danger" of modern-day stress.[9]

Unknowingly, many of us live in a constant fight-or-flight state. We rarely go back into a state of relaxation and rest unless we intentionally do so. That's why it pays to manage stress with the Triple-P strategy: perceive, predict, prepare. The better you get at managing fight-or-flight responses and stress in general, the better you'll protect your health and your well-being from its ravages and the smarter your eating decisions will become.

ARE YOU IN FIGHT-OR-FLIGHT MODE? A FIVE-SECOND STRESS TEST

It's important to stay on top of the physiological clues your body gives you. If you aren't sure how stressed out you are, your body can provide some important clues, and you already have the tools to manage your stress.

Clue: Body temperature.
> *Test:* Clasp your hands. Are they cold? When you're stressed, your blood tends to drain from your extremities. At the same time, your forehead might be sweating.
> *Do:* Try the mindful meditation in chapter 2.

Clue: Muscle tension.
> *Test:* Are your muscles tense?
> *Do:* Consciously relax your muscles using the relax, reboot, release, and recharge exercise described later in this chapter.

Clue: Breathing.
> *Test:* Are you breathing more quickly than normal?
> *Do:* Try the Q-TIPP in chapter 2.

Perceive: Tuning In to Stress

Stress is not a person, a situation, or an event. It's your unique perception of and reaction to a person, situation, or event. Just like beauty, stress is in the eye of the beholder. While some situations or events are universally stressful—caring for an infant or an aging parent, for example—the things that stress you out may roll right off another's back, and vice versa. This is where EI is helpful—you carefully choose how to respond to an event.

I recently witnessed this at my cousin's gymnastic meet. One ten-year-old fell off the balance beam and, unfazed, hopped right back on. She even gave the crowd a wave. The next girl fell off the beam, dissolved into tears, and left the event, her face hidden in her sweatshirt. The same thing occurs in boardrooms; one CEO rants and raves over a financial loss while another shrugs and says, "You win some, you lose some."

But as you've seen, our perception of, and reaction to, stress has a physiological basis. On that level, you can't always consciously perceive the changes occurring in your body. But you can certainly feel their effects. Furthermore, if you monitor what you tell yourself about the stress you're experiencing, you can see some telltale signs that your body is, or has, amped up.

For one, under stress, the urge to eat hits quickly and feels overpowering and all-consuming. My clients tell me things like this:

- "When I'm stressed out, I eat anything that isn't nailed down."
- "When I feel overwhelmed at work, it's either eat the chips or walk out the door, sell my house, and never come back."
- "The kids are driving me nuts. Eating relaxes me and I can handle them better."

I'm betting you can relate. And these examples highlight that powerful physiological reaction, fight or flight, occurring inside you. When you perceive this reaction, you can begin to work with it instead of chalking it up to personal failure or lack of willpower. You'll know that while fight-or-flight mode revs the engine of overeating, *you* decide if you keep your foot on the gas or use the brake. That's EI, and Eat.Q., at work.

When you learn to perceive your level of stress, you can stay on top of it and immediately take steps to alleviate it. Take a look at the following chart. What symptoms of stress are you experiencing right now?

TOO STRESSED TO EAT?

If, while under stress, you turn *away* from food—lose your appetite, even for foods you love, or simply forget to eat—EI skills can still be helpful. In fact, as you read this chapter, substitute the word "overeating" with "undereating" or "not eating."

Though your appetite is gone, your system is still overwhelmed. In freeze mode such as this, it's hard to perceive with accuracy what's going on in your body. If you're losing weight without trying to, mindful meditation (chapter 2) can calm the physiological aspects of stress so you can "hear" your body alerting you to its need for food.

You need to eat, even if you don't feel like it, and on a regular schedule, if possible. You'll keep your energy up and think more clearly.

Predict: Don't Let Stress Shape Your Decisions

In session, Hannah handed her food journal to me with a sigh. "I was doing so well," she lamented.

It was true; the forty-five-year-old accountant had done some excellent work on improving her eating habits. I scanned the food journal in surprise. She listed semidaily stops at a doughnut shop right near her work and more impulse buys at the vending machine.

"I know, I know," Hannah groaned, covering her face. But she didn't know. Not yet.

"Are you experiencing more stress than usual this week?" I asked.

Bingo. It all came pouring out: For the past week Hannah's boss had been under investigation for fraud. While she felt confident that she had done nothing wrong, the office was thick with tension and fear. Hannah and her coworkers knew that the IRS was watching and checking their every move and transaction, and they were *all* under investigation. She was terrified to make even a single mathematical error.

A true professional, Hannah made decisions at work that were still spot-on, even while under considerable stress. But her eating decisions had hit the skids.

The fact is stress affects our ability to make decisions that reflect our best interests. But you don't need to be under investigation to crack under stress.

The day after pulling an all-nighter with a sick child or bidding on a new house, stress starts eroding your ability to make the decisions you would make otherwise.

Studies of the brain show that we are prone to mistakes and have difficulty learning new skills when under stress, but that's not the only reason the quality of our decisions plummets. The biggest reason is the fight-or-flight response, which sends us into freeze, flee, or fight mode. Unfortunately, we focus our decisions around these primitive reactions rather than logic and reason. Second, under stress you are more likely to revert to automatic behaviors that require little thought or effort. Finally, stress affects our perception and experience of the reward value of food.[10]

Even small stresses can negatively affect food decisions, a study conducted at Stanford University shows. In this study, the researchers divided 165

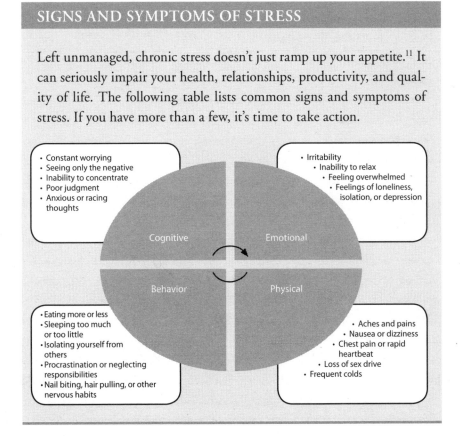

SIGNS AND SYMPTOMS OF STRESS

Left unmanaged, chronic stress doesn't just ramp up your appetite.[11] It can seriously impair your health, relationships, productivity, and quality of life. The following table lists common signs and symptoms of stress. If you have more than a few, it's time to take action.

Cognitive
- Constant worrying
- Seeing only the negative
- Inability to concentrate
- Poor judgment
- Anxious or racing thoughts

Emotional
- Irritability
- Inability to relax
- Feeling overwhelmed
- Feelings of loneliness, isolation, or depression

Behavior
- Eating more or less
- Sleeping too much or too little
- Isolating yourself from others
- Procrastination or neglecting responsibilities
- Nail biting, hair pulling, or other nervous habits

Physical
- Aches and pains
- Nausea or dizziness
- Chest pain or rapid heartbeat
- Loss of sex drive
- Frequent colds

students into two groups. One group was given a two-digit number to re-member as they walked from one room to another. The other group got a seven-digit number. In the second room, they could choose between a slice of chocolate cake and a bowl of fruit salad. The students asked to remember the seven-digit number were nearly twice as likely to choose the cake as those given the two-digit number. It may be that the extra digits overtaxed the stu-dents' brains, the researchers said. In simple terms, when the brain's process-ing resources are tied up (as they are when trying to remember a long number), impulse tends to have a greater impact on your decisions than thought. As a result, you're more likely to choose the option you want—an emotion-driven choice—rather than the one you know is the healthiest choice.[12]

The good news is that even when you're stressed, you can still make solid decisions. Using a mindful pause gives you the opportunity to increase your focus beyond the immediate aspects of a situation in order to take in the information needed to make a good decision. Furthermore, when you add a pause, you can work through your first impulse to say "I can't take it any-more!" and adapt your response.[13]

THE EAT METHOD MODEL OF STRESS EATING

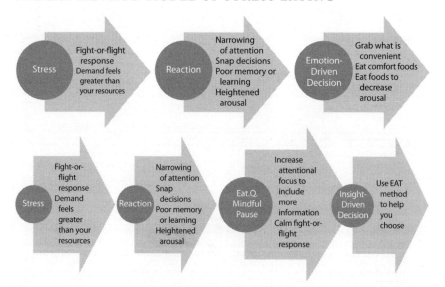

When stress triggers the fight-or-flight response, you can react (let physiology take over) or respond (consciously take steps to manage hyperarousal).

QUIZ: WHAT KIND OF STRESS EATER ARE YOU?

Although everyone knows what stress eating means, it's a generic term that encompasses many feelings. It approaches, but does not capture, how you feel at the moment you choose to use food to feel better. However, to find the right tools to cope, you'll need to dig deeper. This quiz can help you zero in on the specific emotion(s) that make you vulnerable to stress eating.

1. When you are under stress, you . . .

    a. are unable to concentrate. You just can't think straight.

    b. are irritable or think negatively. You focus on the unfairness of an event or situation and are quick to judge and blame.

    c. brood. You obsess about the stressful situation; you can't let it go.

    d. are teary. You cry, seeing the stressful situation as hopeless or insurmountable.

2. When you feel stressed, you typically react by . . .

    a. freezing. You shut down and feel overwhelmed by the situation.

    b. fighting. You yell and want to strike back.

    c. fleeing. You want to run away from the situation because it makes you intensely uncomfortable.

    d. feeling a combination or all of the above, depending on the situation.

3. Stress tends to hit you in the . . .

    a. mind. You feel like a hamster in a cage: no matter how fast you spin, you never get anywhere.

    b. body. You express your stress with gestures or vocals—you put your hands up as a warning sign, put them over your face, maybe even grunt or moan. Your body feels tense, or you get a headache.

    c. stomach. You feel like you want to throw up. You pace the floor, sweating and holding your stomach, your heart pounding.

    d. soul. You feel crushed. You just want to lie on the sofa and not move. You're unmotivated, tired, and tearful.

4. It's late at night, and finally the house is quiet. It's been a long day. A thought pops into your mind: *I'm gonna eat.* Which thought is likely to precede that one?

    a. *I'm so tired. I've had a tough day.*

    b. *I'm so irritated. I can't stand this.*

    c. *I'm at the end of my rope. I know I need to unwind, but how?*

    d. *I'm so done. I just can't cope anymore.*

5. Your boss pokes her head into your office and assigns you yet another task to be completed by the end of the day. You haven't even finished yesterday's projects. Your first thought is . . .

    a. *This is just too, too much.*

    b. *That witch. She just keeps piling it on.*

    c. *Oh my god, oh my god, oh my god . . .*

    d. *I give up. I just give up. There's no one to help, and no one cares.*

SCORING

If you chose mainly (a) answers, you stress eat in response to feeling overwhelmed. If you chose mainly (b) answers, your stress eating is fueled by anger.

If you chose mainly (c) answers, anxiety drives your stress eating. If you chose mainly (d) answers, you eat in response to feeling sadness or loneliness.

If your answers didn't reveal a distinct pattern, you may stress eat in response to any or all of the emotions above. This means that you'll really have to pause in the moment and think about the *exact* feeling triggering you to eat. Once you know what feeling makes you most vulnerable to stress-driven eating, you can watch for it. With patience and practice, you'll increase your ability to diagnose that feeling, press PAUSE, and make an insight-driven decision.

Prepare: Relax, Reboot, Release, and Recharge

"When I'm stressed, everything I know about healthy eating goes out the window!" I've heard this from clients countless times, and I get it. The urge to eat is so strong it feels difficult to respond in any other manner. But while it feels hard, it's less so if you have a plan in place for those must-eat moments.

When you hear your mind say *Stop!* you've hit a red flag—a signal that you've reached a moment of decision specifically around stress eating. The Four Rs can help get you through it:

PEEL AWAY YOUR STRESS

I don't recommend eating when you are stressed—that creates a strong connection in the brain that when you feel stress, you eat. But if you are stressed and feel that you *must* eat, try a clementine orange.[14] Naturally sweet, without a drop of added sugar, they're also seedless (who wants to deal with seeds when they're stressed?) and easy to throw in your bag and take with you.

In this self-soothing exercise, a blend of mindfulness and stress reduction, you'll use the process of peeling one of these fragrant beauties to temporarily distract yourself from whatever is bothering you.

- Slowly unpeel the clementine. As you peel, focus on the process of peeling—how easily the fruit slips away from the skin, the bumps and ripples on the skin, the strong scent that is released as you peel.

- Pick up a piece of the peel and squeeze gently; take a deep whiff. The smell of citrus is naturally calming.

- Savor one segment at a time. If you typically crave sweets when you're stressed, tune in to the natural sweetness.

Two clementines have a day's worth of vitamin C,[15] which helps boost your immune system, which is compromised by stress. So if you want another, go ahead!

Step 1: Relax. To switch off the fight-or-flight response, do any one of the keep-calm tools in chapter 2. Or try *progressive muscle relaxation,* a stress-management technique in which you tighten and then release specific muscle groups from your head to your toes. It's one of my favorites because it's so simple to do. Relaxing your muscles can help your mind relax. Simply find a quiet place and take a few moments to breathe slowly and deeply. When you feel relaxed, start with your right foot. Squeeze the muscles as tightly as you can and hold for a count of ten. Relax your right foot and take a few deep breaths. Then repeat with your left foot. Slowly work your way up

TO LOWER YOUR CORTISOL, RAISE YOUR AWARENESS

"The best way out is always through," to quote the poet Robert Frost. Stress eating is like taking an emotional detour around the feeling. Mindfulness can help you tunnel right through stress and emerge on the other side of it. In a study conducted at the University of California at San Francisco, simple mindful eating and stress-reduction techniques helped prevent weight gain—and without dieting.

The study participants—all women, all chronically stressed, and either overweight or obese—were not put on diets. Instead, twenty-four of the women were randomly assigned to mindfulness training and practice. The remaining twenty-three served as a control group.

The women in the mindfulness training group were taught stress-reduction techniques that included mindful yoga stretches and several types of meditations, including a mindfulness meditation technique called the body scan. They were also led through guided meditations that introduced mindful eating practices such as paying attention to body sensations, for example, hunger, fullness, taste satisfaction, and food cravings. This group was also encouraged to practice mindful eating during their meals and meditation exercises thirty minutes a day.

All the participants took a chronic stress inventory to gauge their levels of psychological stress before the four-month study began and again after it was over. The researchers also monitored the women's

your body—legs, belly, back, chest, arms, neck, face—squeezing and relaxing each group of muscles.[16] The contrast between squeezing and relaxing reduces stress and feels rejuvenating.

Step 2: Reboot. As we've discussed, stress is linked to your perception of events. Under stress, faced with the decision to eat or not, reboot your mind to focus on what you *can* do rather than what you *can't*. If you're thinking *I just can't help stress eating,* welcome in that feeling. Then counter it with *I have lots of choices.* And you do. You can choose to walk away from the food, toss the cookies in the bin, opt for a healthier meal or snack, save the food for

---

percentages of body fat in general and abdominal fat specifically, as well as their cortisol levels, measuring secretion of the hormone shortly after the women awakened.

Cortisol levels typically rise when a person wakes up in the morning. But threats—real or perceived—also trigger cortisol secretion. If we wake up dreading a stressful day ahead, cortisol may rise even higher.

The study found that among women in the treatment group, those who showed the most improvements in perceiving their bodies' cues, or greater reductions in stress or cortisol, lost the most abdominal fat. Simply put, the greater the women's reduction in stress, the more belly fat they lost.

Among the subset of obese women, those who'd received mindfulness training showed significant reductions in morning cortisol and also maintained their total body weight. By comparison, the cortisol levels of the women in the control group didn't change, and those women continued to gain weight.

The study's findings suggest you can train your mind to notice, but not to automatically react to, habitual patterns—to not unthinkingly head for food when you're angry or stressed, for example. If you can recognize what you are feeling in the moment, *before* you act, you're more likely to make a healthier choice.

later, and so forth. When you reboot, you face the moment of decision with a fresh perspective, that of a person with choices.

Step 3: Release. The ability to let go is a critical stress-management skill. Most often, the struggle and pain of stress is rooted in holding on to a negative feeling or idea. When you let go, you accept that in this moment, stress or no stress, life is unfolding exactly as it should. When your mind struggles against a stressful situation—typically by brooding or obsessing over how unjust it is—counter that negative chatter. Repeat silently, *Let it go,* until your mind releases the struggle. If you're a visual type, you might imagine yourself holding on to a branch sticking out from the edge of a cliff, letting go of that tree branch, and dropping safely into life as it is.

Step 4: Recharge. You can't pour from a jug that is empty, or so the saying goes. Stress can make you feel empty, causing you to want to fill up with food instead of with other enriching activities. You need a way to recharge your batteries by filling up on something besides food. In moments like this, call or e-mail someone; connecting can fill the emptiness and recharge your emotional battery. So too can a nap, deep breathing, a walk in the woods, or a half hour of knitting or other crafts.

The Four Rs are easy to remember (especially when you're feeling overwhelmed) and simple to do, and they really work. If you do them faithfully, you'll learn that you don't have to reach for food when you feel overwhelmed, and you don't have to let your mind convince you that you have no other options. The Four Rs help you find them.

Design Your Customized Triple-P Plan

Managing stress starts with a healthy lifestyle: getting enough sleep; maintaining a healthy diet; limiting alcohol, nicotine, caffeine, and other substances; regularly exercising to blow off steam. The irony is that when you're constantly under the gun, these good habits fall by the wayside. But there's a way out: creating your own customized Triple-P plan.

The following example can get you started. But because your stressors are unique to you, the solutions to those stressors—and the overeating they trigger—come from within.

RED FLAG

I Typically Stress Eat When I'm Angry or Irritated

In a good moment: I call a friend to distract myself, blow off steam by going on a run, or engage in some positive self-talk.

In a difficult moment: I have a meltdown, snap at anyone around me, maybe even throw a tantrum, and crunch through a bag of crisps.

TRIPLE-P PLAN

I can *perceive* by . . . paying close attention to the physiological and cognitive signs of anger. For me, the signs are irrational thoughts, such as *It doesn't matter anyway,* or even vengeful thoughts, such as *I'll show* him *what I will and won't do.* My other red flags: I feel hot, have trouble focusing, and brood on the situation.

I can *predict* by . . . being mindful that anger clouds the rational part of my brain. I try not to make any decisions until I've cooled off. This means choosing an amount of time—it may be five minutes or five hours, depending on how high my anger level is.

I can *prepare* by . . . not venting my anger. Research has found that venting—punching a pillow, going on a full-bore rant—can sometimes fuel the fire by increasing your blood pressure and your adrenaline level as you talk.[17] It's true for me; I can get really fired up. Instead, the key for me is to defuse the anger with the tools in chapter 2. I also find ways to literally cool down: get a cold drink, change into a short-sleeved shirt, or turn on the air conditioning.

Ready to give it a try? Read through the following common stressors. Pick the one that derails your eating most often, or write a different one that's unique to you. Then fill in the blanks to create a Triple-P plan. For ideas and inspiration, use the Four Rs, the suggestions in the box on page 186, and the tools in chapter 2.

RED FLAG

I Typically Stress Eat When I'm Overwhelmed or Overextended

In a good moment:

_____

_____

In a difficult moment:

_____

_____

TRIPLE-P PLAN

I can *perceive* by . . .

_____

_____

_____

I can *predict* by . . .

_____

_____

_____

I can *prepare* by . . .

_____

_____

_____

I Typically Stress Eat When I'm Upset by Conflicts with My Partner, Family, or Coworkers

In a good moment:

_____

_____

In a difficult moment:

_____

_____

TRIPLE-P PLAN

I can *perceive* by . . .

_____

_____

_____

I can *predict* by . . .

_____

_____

_____

I can *prepare* by . . .

_____

_____

_____

STRESS AND DECISION MAKING: IDENTIFYING YOUR LEVEL OF URGENCY

There's a strong link between what you feel and your decision to engage in stress eating. If you press PAUSE and perceive that your thoughts are pushing you toward food, you have time to stage a successful "intervention."

In the following examples, ponder the emotions associated with the words *must, need, want,* and *obsessed.* As you'll see in tool 18 (page 269), these small words have an inordinate amount of power to shape the way you think, which affects the decisions you make.

Code Red: *That's it! I* must *eat to save my sanity!*
Intervention: Minimize the damage.

At this point, it's likely that you feel unable to pull yourself away, and you're probably in the middle of emotionally driven eating. Normally, I don't advise eating when you're stressed, but even if you're at Code Red, you can still consciously choose healthier foods—rather than chomping on crisps, try carrots and hummus. Do a mindfulness exercise to calm down. Just do the best you can to calm down your stress response, which is likely on hyperalert! After this incident, debrief and write in your Eat.Q. notebook all the behavioral, psychological, physical, and cognitive factors that led up to this moment. It's likely that this incident, or one like it, will happen again. You can predict it and be prepared for the next time.

Code Orange: *I'm about to blow. I* need *food to feel better.*
Intervention: Expand your options.

It's likely at this juncture that the urge is pretty strong. Look closely at the T tools and find at least one other choice. Reframe the word "need" in your mind to "choice." This puts the power and control back in your hands instead of making it like a biological need, such as the need to breathe or eat.

Code Yellow: *I'm overwhelmed and I* want *chocolate!*
Intervention: Steer this desire in a different direction.

> You know what you're feeling. You've identified the food craving and the emotions. At this point, overeating still feels like a choice or a desire, not a done deal. Try to match your feeling with what you do. If you feel sad, cry or call someone. If you're tired, sleep.

Code Green: *I'm exhausted and irritable, and* obsessed *with thoughts of chocolate.*
Intervention: Stay the course.

> You perceive the urge to stress eat. Good for you! Don't judge yourself. That urge is natural, and obsessing about chocolate isn't eating it. Accept that you're obsessing, and use that insight to turn to a non-food alternative—perhaps a mindfulness exercise?—to cool your stress.

> Now that you're tuned in to your biological response to stress, you must predict your next move.

Brooke's Stress Makeover

When I began my psychology career, client files were still on paper. Even before I met clients face to face, I used the thickness of their files as a rule of thumb: thick files nearly always correlated with stress-related symptoms. Brooke is a great example of a thick-file client who used the EAT method to help her learn to stay one step ahead of her stress level.

Brooke, a fifty-five-year-old substance-abuse counselor, was a former flower child who favored Indian-print skirts and scarves and wore her gray-blonde hair down her back. I often get referrals from doctors when they can't find a physical cause to a health problem, and Brooke came to me with a number of vague complaints—fatigue, mild depression, weight gain. Her doctor had run tests, prescribed antidepressants, and ordered blood work,

without effect. She also suffered from frequent headaches and had lost her
sex drive. Her husband was beginning to take her lack of interest personally.

After several sessions of discussing her symptoms and eating patterns,
I diagnosed her with caregiver burnout. A veteran counselor—she'd been
on the job for thirty years—Brooke was dedicated to her clients and had
a heavy caseload. She took newbie counselors under her wing and worked

FOODS THAT BUFFER THE EFFECTS OF STRESS

While the urge to eat when you feel stressed is in part biological, research suggests that certain vitamins and minerals can help calm the
body and soothe the ravages of stress. If you have a stressful and busy
life, the foods below can help make you less vulnerable to the effects
of stress.

1. *Dark chocolate* helps release dopamine, a brain chemical associ-
    ated with pleasure.[18] It's helpful to mindfully savor one ounce a
    day, the recommended daily amount.

2. *Oatmeal* is rich in complex carbohydrates, involved in the release
    of serotonin. This brain chemical, which plays a major role in
    the regulation of mood and appetite, helps keep cravings in
    check.[19]

3. *Kiwi* is an excellent source of vitamin C, which boosts the
    immune system and reduces cortisol levels.[20] This is important
    because your immune system is compromised when stressed and
    makes you more susceptible to illness. Other C-rich foods include
    guavas, bell peppers, oranges, papaya, and strawberries.

4. *Spinach* is rich in the mineral magnesium, which plays a key role
    in regulating and lowering blood pressure[21] (blood pressure is
    often raised by stress). Enjoy it as a salad, add to pasta, or slide a
    few leaves into a sandwich.

5. *Skimmed milk* contains tryptophan, an amino acid that creates
    serotonin and that research has linked with making people feel

with the toughest addicts—the "frequent fliers" who dropped in and out of treatment. She wrapped her kindness and compassion in a gravelly I-mean-business, don't-pull-any-crap voice honed from decades of working with addicts and alcoholics.

In her younger days, she could leave the stress of her job at work. Now she tossed and turned in bed, worrying about her clients. Unable to sleep, Brooke

relaxed[22] and sleepy. Try a glass if you can't sleep or to help reduce stress-related PMS symptoms.

6. *Salmon* is rich in healthy fats called omega-3 fatty acids, which reduce inflammation and pain.[23] To ramp down your stress level, eat foods that can help reduce pain and swelling. If you don't like salmon, try walnuts, flaxseed, cabbage, cauliflower, or omega-3-fortified eggs, milk, juice, and yogurt.

7. *Black tea* contains antioxidants and amino acids that have been found to affect neurotransmitters in the brain. These neurotransmitters naturally reduce levels[24] of the stress hormone cortisol, the hormone that makes you crave sugary, fatty foods.

8. *Avocados* contain healthy monounsaturated fat, which keeps you more satisfied and helps regulate nerve communication, which helps you think clearer.[25] Cut it into slices and put some on a sandwich or just have some for a snack. Or make it into guacamole.

9. *Tart cherries* appear to possess antioxidant and anti-inflammatory properties that help the prevention, treatment, and recovery of soft tissue injury and pain.[26]

10. *Pistachios*, which contain the least amount of fat and calories of any nut, help keep your mood stable and your blood sugar steady.[27] Buy them in the shell—opening them one by one helps you eat them slowly and avoid eating too many.

spent her nights eating—ice cream, biscuits, pizza left over from dinner. Exhausted (and stuffed) in the morning, she'd skip breakfast and rush to work. When she finally got hungry, she'd grab a doughnut; the agency bought dozens for the staff each morning, and the coffee was always brewing.

Brooke's insomnia, the result of the chronic hyperarousal of her stress response, was a classic symptom of caregiver burnout. So was her uncontrolled eating. Although she knew how to lose weight and eat well, the pressure she was under drove her food choices, which were typically based on convenience and comfort.

Learning to use a Triple-P plan turned things around for Brooke. It showed her how to devise better ways to cope with her emotion-driven eating and taught a veteran caregiver to identify, accept, and meet her own needs.

Brooke's Triple-P Plan

While Brooke was quick to perceive her stress, accepting that she didn't know how to fix it proved more challenging. She was a counselor, for goodness sake! She could handle anything! The problem, she soon discovered, was her belief that she *should* be able to handle everything.

The child of alcoholics, Brooke cared for her mother and younger siblings until her late teens, when she left home. She'd always used food to stuff down her fear, anxiety, and anger. In her teens, she turned to drugs and alcohol. Fortunately, she found recovery and dedicated her life to helping fellow addicts and alcoholics.

Brooke uncovered another poignant truth: subconsciously she believed she wouldn't live past age fifty. Not coincidentally, her father had died at fifty, from alcoholism. When you believe you'll die young, like a parent has, why bother to eat well or meet your own physical and emotional needs?

But as we continued our work, Brooke saw that she wanted to live, and although she'd escaped using drugs and alcohol, her unmanaged stress could cut her life short. Our work helped her see and accept the connection between her neglect- and abuse-filled childhood, her chronic stress, and her physical symptoms, including her overeating.

Here's the Triple-P plan Brooke came up with:

Too Many Clients, Not Enough Time

In a good moment:

"I can talk myself through it, with a little bit of sarcasm. I tell myself this stress is a piece of cake compared to some of the stuff I've been through, and a doughnut won't do a damn thing to fix anything."

In a difficult moment:

"I say, 'What the hell. We all die anyway, some sooner than later. If I'm digging my grave with a fork, I'll make it a dessert fork, not a salad fork.'"

TRIPLE-P PLAN

I can *perceive* by . . .

noticing when I'm upset. I start swearing under my breath and shoving files around on my desk. Since I'm good at noticing what other people are feeling—a slight raise of an eyebrow or a quiver in someone's voice—I can imagine that I am my own client. I can ask myself what my body language is telling me right now. If I can't sleep, I can take a hot bath.

I can *predict* by . . .

validating my feelings. I tend to dismiss how I feel. When I hear myself trying to shut down my feelings with *It doesn't really matter* or *You're being a drama queen; keep it together,* I need to snap to attention.

I can *prepare* by . . .

doing what I tell my clients to do: *relax!* Before I go to bed, I can do some deep breathing and meditation to help let go.

I worked with Brooke for years and watched this tough-as-nails survivor start practicing what she preached. In fact, true to her caring and irrepressible nature, she also began to teach her new skills—occasional, informal classes in yoga, journaling, meditation, and healthy eating—on her own time and free to any of the agency's clients. The process of eating healthy and losing weight was slow—it takes time to recover from a life of chronic stress—but her headaches stopped, her sex drive woke up, and she now sleeps through the night. Five years after I first opened her thick folder, she's free.

The Last Bite

Isn't it a relief to know that your desire to eat in moments of stress isn't a personal failure, but normal and natural? That awareness gives you *power*. The next time your boss is demanding, the kids are whiny, or the bills are mounting, you'll know that a cupcake isn't the answer, because you'll have learned to press PAUSE. Once you learn to relax, reboot, and recharge, and design your Triple-P plan, you will feel less out of control and powerless and will see that stress can be managed—without food.

8

Trauma

Note: This chapter discusses emotional traumas of all kinds, and its content may be triggering. If you've experienced trauma that you're still working through, skip it until you feel emotionally ready.

Anything that's human is mentionable, and anything that is mentionable can be more manageable. When we can talk about our feelings, they become less overwhelming, less upsetting, and less scary.

—Fred Rogers

In life, bad things happen, horrible things—the loss of a child, a sudden death, violent crime, sexual abuse, natural disasters. Such events are traumas, emotional earthquakes that can reduce a person's life, and their beliefs about the world, to rubble.

food for THOUGHT

- Have you experienced an event you consider harmful, surprising, or life-altering?
- Do certain images, sounds, or odors upset you or remind you of incidents from the past?
- Do you shut down when upset, or can you share your feelings with those you love and trust?
- When you're distressed, do you eat to numb out or calm down?
- Do you ever feel disconnected from your body, as if what is happening to you is happening to someone else?

After a trauma, some people experience the common stages of grief, including shock, anger, and sadness. At the end of the cycle, they come to an acceptance of their feelings. Others, however, don't experience such resolution. Instead, their feelings become what I call *blocked, blurred,* or *ballooned* (more about these later)—numbed out, confused, or exaggerated. Emotional intelligence can help you acknowledge with compassion this skewing of your feelings.

I see many clients who've experienced trauma, whether recent or long past. But it isn't the emotional earthquake that brings them to my door. It's the emotional effects of that original trauma—what I call *emotional aftershocks.*

My clients believe they've begun counseling to lose weight or manage their overeating, but often the real reason—buried under forty or seventy-five or a hundred and fifty pounds—is that they've experienced trauma in their past, and they are now dealing with the aftershocks.

Maria came to me to lose forty pounds for her daughter's wedding. She'd been an overweight child, and in adulthood she'd lost and regained weight many times. This time, she couldn't lose. In fact, she'd gained a few pounds.

In time, we dug into the rubble of her past. At age ten, Maria lost her father suddenly to an aggressive form of cancer. Her mother, perhaps traumatized herself, reacted to this devastating loss with silence—not a tear, not a hug, not a word. Maria's memories of the loss, and the years after, were spotty. She sank into a quiet darkness and began to eat sugary, fatty foods, which offered her the comfort her mother couldn't.

Seared into her memory, however, was the aftershock: her subsequent weight gain and the taunting she endured from other children, which continued into school. Forty years later, she could tell me the first and last names of her bullies, and still heard their whispers as she passed: "Jelly roll." "Pig." The trauma had frozen her in time. In her mind, she still felt like a fat, lonely, despised little girl who'd suffered a devastating loss.

As we talked, her father's death—long excised from her conscious thought—boiled to the surface. She described her mother's non-reaction as if the loss had happened to someone else—a character in a movie, perhaps. This numbness was a sign of *dissociation,* a protective mechanism called up by the nervous system when it can't handle any more stimulation, so you detach from the physical or emotional sensations that you're experiencing.

Basically, Maria had gone offline emotionally. Although sharing an intensely painful memory, she couldn't feel it, couldn't experience it.

I shared this observation with her. And then came . . . tears—warm, salty, human tears. She tried to stop them and couldn't. No one had ever validated her devastation at her father's death, asked her if she wanted to talk about it, urged her to cry. Now, as she *felt* the loss, *understood* the connection between her uncontrolled eating and her sudden, excruciating loss, she could begin to heal.

The fear, horror, and other intense, negative feelings unleashed by a traumatic event can bury people beneath its rubble, leaving them unable to cope with the feelings related to the aftershocks. Dissociation allows their bodies to run on autopilot. Food is the misguided consolation of aftershock, its numbing powers burying the unbearable, unspeakable past beneath protective layers of weight.

A trauma aftershock is the mind's attempt to protect you and to reregulate your emotions. But if you never move past it, the protection turns to destruction. A helpful way to heal from emotional trauma is to understand and articulate the feelings you've buried and develop skills to cope with them that don't involve food.

Basically, you've got to dig, as Maria was ultimately able to do. With therapy, she came to understand that she no longer had to push down her feelings with food. She could express those feelings, because it was now safe to do so. You can too. This chapter explores how trauma can alter feelings, thereby affecting emotional intelligence, and how to use, understand, and integrate the feelings around the trauma to heal its aftershocks, including overeating.

Trauma: More Common than You Think

Maybe you're thinking that you've had rough periods in your life. But could you really call your "rough times" trauma?

It's not only possible; it's probable. Most of us are exposed to at least one traumatic situation in our lives, research shows,[1] and such experiences can have a profound impact on your weight and eating.

Trauma is any extraordinarily stressful event or situation that shatters your sense of security. Often traumas are not within your power to prevent, which leaves you feeling helpless and vulnerable. Examples of traumatic experiences include natural disasters or accidents; physical, emotional, or sexual abuse; alcoholism or drug abuse (your own or a family member's); childhood neglect or bullying; and physical illnesses, surgeries, car accidents, job loss, divorce, and disabilities (your own or a family member's).[2]

Trauma is not one-size-fits-all; what makes a situation or an event a trauma

PTSD: NOT LIMITED TO SOLDIERS

Left untreated, blocked, blurred, or ballooned feelings caused by traumatic experiences may snowball into post-traumatic stress disorder (PTSD).[3] Essentially, this anxiety disorder changes or damages the fight-or-flight response, and people who have it feel stressed or afraid even when they're no longer in danger.[4]

PTSD is often associated with combat veterans. However, I've treated countless men and women who developed it after physical or sexual assault, abuse, accidents, or disasters; after the sudden loss of a loved one; or after a friend or family member experienced danger or was harmed. Its symptoms are typically grouped into three categories:[5]

- *Reliving the Trauma.* Flashbacks—reliving the trauma over and over, including physical symptoms, such as a racing heart or sweating—are common. You may also relive the trauma in nightmares about the event.

- *Hyperarousal.* You may be easily startled, feel tense or on edge, find it hard to sleep, and/or have angry outbursts. The stress and anger that accompany hyperarousal can make it hard to sleep, eat, or concentrate, and you may use alcohol or drugs to soothe or calm yourself.

- *Avoidance and Isolation.* You may avoid people, places, or things that remind you of the trauma. When you do encounter these reminders, you may experience flashbacks.

is the way you experience it and your reaction to it. For example, two of my acquaintances were in a car accident together. Though the car was totaled, both walked away with only bumps and bruises. One got behind the wheel right away. The other developed severe panic and stopped driving altogether. Same trauma; very different reactions.

Symptoms that may be caused by trauma include:[6]

- *Psychological Distress.* You may feel sadness, fear, anxiety or agitation, anger, horror, and grief.

- *Numbness.* Initially you may be in shock and feel "shut down."

- *Depression.* You may feel a pervasive sense of sadness, have crying spells, and experience feelings of helplessness and pessimism. You may lose interest in your usual activities and find it difficult to concentrate.

- *Confusion.* You may have very intense feelings but be unable to identify them or put them into words.

- *Physical Symptoms.* These include insomnia or sleeping too much, lack of interest in sex, lack of energy, and pain with no apparent cause.

Other signs and symptoms of trauma include an inability to trust, a fear of taking risks, feelings of worthlessness, and thoughts of suicide in the extreme.[7]

The Trauma–Eating Connection

The connection between trauma and eating problems seems simple: overeating or other eating issues develop as a way to cope with overwhelming or painful feelings prompted by the trauma, or as a bid to gain control over the trauma and the emotions it causes.

As a psychologist, I can tell you that making that connection can be anything but simple. A new client may be focused on a "fast-food addiction," and it can take weeks or months to trace it to a trauma that occurred one, ten, or even thirty years before. Remember, it's not the trauma itself that manifests in disordered eating. It's the way of coping with the feeling produced by the trauma. The following are a few examples from my practice that help show the connection between trauma and eating issues.

COULD YOU BE BLOCKED, BLURRED, OR BALLOONED?

After a trauma, emotions can become blocked (numbed out), blurred (confused), or ballooned (exaggerated). As you read, see which category seems to fit your experience of your feelings.

Blocked

____ numbness

____ robotic behavior—"going through the motions"

____ disconnection from an experience (for example, feeling as if you're watching yourself in a movie)

____ discussion of the traumatic experience as if it happened to someone else

Blurred

____ memories from the past pop up in the present

____ triggers create feelings that don't make sense in the current context (for example, you jump when your mobile phone rings)

____ oversensitivity to current triggers

____ nightmares

____ exaggerated responses—over- or under-responding

Ballooned

____ hyperarousal and/or overalertness to danger

____ difficulty sleeping, eating and/or concentrating

____ oversensitivity

____ rapid breathing

Loneliness equals overeating. One of my clients was raised by her mother after a bitter divorce, and the loss of income forced her mother to work long hours. My client spent each afternoon after school at her grandparents' house, where her grandmother fed her cookies and extra meals. Their house was so warm and loving, unlike her lonely, empty home. She loved sitting with her grandmother at the kitchen table chatting after school. As an adult, in times of loneliness, she found food to be her sole comfort.

Self-loathing and guilt equal restricting, bingeing, purging. In school, a male client received after-school tutoring from an extremely popular teacher. One day during their lesson, the male teacher sexually assaulted him. Ashamed and embarrassed, my client was terrified to tell anyone. No one would believe him, he feared. People would think he was gay. No girl would date him, and the guys would beat him up. At first he quit eating, so strong was his anxiety that the incident would be discovered. Later, however, his guilt, shame, and self-loathing led him to restrict what he ate to regain the control over his body his teacher had taken from him. Eventually he began starving, binge-ing, and purging. Purging, in particular, gave him a great sense of relief; his anxiety melted away instantly, as if he were vomiting out all his fear and anger about the assault.

Anger equals bingeing. One of my clients worked two jobs for almost ten years to put her husband through medical school. In the first month of her husband's new residency, he had an affair with a surgeon from the hospi-tal. Fury consumed every part of my client's being. However, in her family "ladies" didn't get angry.

She found that eating worked to push the anger deep inside her, and she gained more and more weight. Each time the anger threatened to surface, a food craving popped up. Satisfying it pushed the anger back down again. Her compulsive eating wasn't just a cover for her anger; it also served to punish her for feeling "stupid" and "unworthy."

In the face of these types of overwhelming experiences and feelings, it's understandable why you turn to food to cope. The way out, ironically, is to go in. When you confront the trauma in your life and accept that it happened, you've taken the first critical steps to establishing a healthier relationship with food.

Emotional Earthquakes Rock Emotional Intelligence

While trauma is a normal reaction to abnormal situations, traumatic experiences send the nervous system into overdrive. This hyperarousal of the nervous system moves your body into a state of chronic stress (chapter 7), which weakens your ability to regulate your emotions.

People who have experienced trauma often have trouble knowing what they are feeling; understanding where these feelings come from and why they have them; using their feelings to live in a healthy, positive way; or managing feelings so they don't affect their jobs, relationships, or weight. Trauma does a number on these very abilities, which are the hallmarks of emotional intelligence.

I describe the connection between trauma and EI to my clients using the metaphor of mirrors. If you look into a full-length mirror, your image is reflected back to you exactly as it is, from head to toe. If you look into a compact mirror, you see one small part of yourself, perhaps just your lips or one eye. And when you see yourself in a fun-house mirror, you see a warped and distorted image of yourself.

Trauma is the emotional equivalent of a fun-house mirror: it distorts and twists feelings. Your emotions may be magnified, or you may dissociate. In short, it's difficult or impossible to trust those feelings. If your emotions are at either end of the extreme—either hypervigilant or cut off—it may be difficult to remain calm or calm down. Extreme difficulty self-regulating emotions as a result of trauma can sometimes lead to eating disorders, along with PTSD.

Worse is if you manage to express your feelings and someone close to you does not validate them. If you've been in a car accident, it can be devastating to hear your partner or a friend say that your reluctance to get behind the wheel or to ride as a passenger is "silly." If you've been the victim of sexual abuse and hear a relative who doesn't know about it speak highly of the perpetrator, you may lose trust in your feelings or doubt your sanity.

To heal from trauma, it's essential to understand that your feelings are not a perfect reflection of your natural state. They are a normal reaction to an abnormal event. When intense feelings related to the trauma are triggered (you hear a voice like your ex-husband's or you see a child on TV with cancer), it's important to ask yourself if your strong reaction is a result of the way the incident is being reflected back to you.

THE EAT METHOD MODEL OF TRAUMA

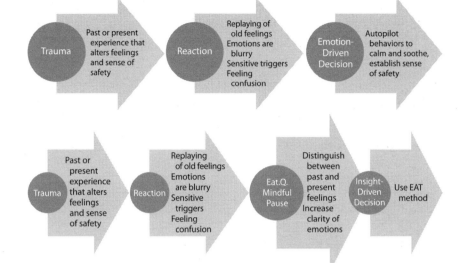

Trauma can alter your feelings, making them more intense, disconnecting you from them, or triggering feelings from the past in the present. This makes it difficult to have feelings that match your current experience. A mindful pause helps you reevaluate the feelings to determine whether they could be skewed by trauma.

The Trauma–Eating Connection

Only soldiers in active combat "get" PTSD, right? Wrong. Not only is this life-rending malady an equal-opportunity disorder, but also its roots are often in childhood trauma. Several clinical and community studies have associated exposure to childhood abuse and early-life stress with a higher risk for obesity.[8]

Think about the message on every passenger-door mirror. On it is etched the words OBJECTS IN MIRROR ARE CLOSER THAN THEY APPEAR. It's human nature to want distressing or even horrifying experiences to be far from our conscious thoughts and experiences. For example, if you experienced childhood neglect or abuse, a natural disaster, or an acrimonious breakup, you would prefer it be long behind you, even though it feels raw and close. But these experiences aren't far away; they're just below the surface, or dormant and awaiting a trigger to awaken them. When these experiences feel too close, they cause tremendous pain. This is why people who have experienced trauma often push away feelings with food.

Research bears this out. In a 2012 study, researchers at the University of Massachusetts Medical School in Worcester collected data from the Collaborative Psychiatric Epidemiology Surveys (CPES), which comprise three national studies of 20,013 men and women conducted between 2001 and 2003. Among those with PTSD diagnosed in the year before they participated in the study, nearly one-third (32.6 percent) were obese, compared to less than one-quarter of those with no history of PTSD (24.1 percent).[9] That's even after researchers factored in depression, substance and alcohol abuse or dependence, and other variables. There was no difference between men and women.

KNOW YOUR TRIGGERS

One of my former clients, Anna, lost her home in a flood. The rain fell swiftly and before she knew it, she was trapped on the roof of her home. Thankfully, she and her loved ones survived, but every possession she owned was carried away before her eyes.

Anna's feeling of safety and security had been permanently altered. After the flood, rain or even a cloudy sky triggered memories of the devastating loss of her home and caused extreme anxiety. The two things that calmed her were watching the Weather Channel all day and eating.

Memories of the traumatic event can invade your consciousness at any time. You may feel as if you're reliving the event and experiencing the same fear and horror. This is called a *flashback*. Sometimes flashbacks are preceded by a *trigger*—a sound or sight that "returns" you to the event. For a woman who was sexually assaulted, seeing a news report of a rape may trigger a flashback, or a crash survivor may experience a flashback while witnessing an accident.[11]

You may try to avoid triggering situations or people that bring the past into your present, or refuse to talk or think about the event. For example, if you were robbed at gunpoint while working at a burger place, you may avoid all fast-food restaurants.[12]

However, avoiding triggers is an exhausting way to live, and it limits

While the link between PTSD and obesity isn't entirely clear, the study noted that PTSD is associated with alterations in the function of the HPA axis, the hormonal system that activates the fight-or-flight response. The HPA axis regulates cortisol secretion. Studies have linked abnormally high cortisol levels to stress-related weight gain and increases and decreases in food intake induced by stress.

Another possibility is that a deficit in *inhibitory control* plays a part in the PTSD–obesity link. Inhibitory control includes abilities such as the capacity to think before you act, pay attention despite distractions, and act

your life. It's just as important to realize that the control you seek is an illusion. The solution is to familiarize yourself with your triggers. When you know what they are, you can be ready for them and take positive, self-soothing actions to help regulate the feelings of fear, horror, and helplessness they can call up.

If you don't think you have triggers, or don't know what they are, enlist the help of a trusted friend or therapist to bring them to the surface. In Anna's case, she noticed that some days she felt fine while others made her extremely anxious. As we discussed it, she had an insight: her anxiety was linked to looking out a window. Unconsciously, she had been scanning the sky for signs of rain. If the sky looked dark, she ate more to calm herself.

If you've experienced trauma, learning to identify your triggers is a key aspect of making insight-driven decisions. These days, if Anna begins to munch mindlessly, she understands that her memories of the flood may have been triggered, and she uses a keep-calm tool (chapter 2) to quell her anxiety. She might repeat a soothing affirmation, such as "I am a strong person and a survivor." She may head to her craft table and her scrapbooking projects. And each day she scans the sky. If it's dark, she reminds herself that floods are rare and that the forecasters know in advance that they're coming.

appropriately when tempted to do otherwise.[12] When people with PTSD are given tasks that measure inhibitory control, they tend to perform poorly, the study noted. Recent research suggests that inhibitory control is a must-have in order for someone to pass up the abundance of pleasurable food in our environment. Supporting this notion are findings that link deficits in inhibitory control to obesity and poor weight-loss outcomes in behavioral treatment programs.

Overall, the University of Massachusetts findings jibe with what I see in my clients who have experienced trauma. Some lose their desire to eat for a time. But if they cannot or will not confront the traumatic event, the desire to eat often comes roaring back. Locked deep in a troubled heart, painful, frightening, and even horrifying memories drive them to high-fat, high-sugar comfort foods to help them numb out. The trouble is that food—even pleasurable food—cannot quell pain this deep. The feeling of fullness doesn't last for long, and the hunger will return, unless the memories and emotions are dealt with eventually.

When Trauma Steals Your Voice

People who experience trauma can lose more than their sense of self or their understanding of and trust in the world. Compounding such losses is the loss of their ability to understand and express their feelings—the alexithymia (the inability to put your feelings into words) we discussed in chapter 3.

I often see clients with extreme alexithymia. Many have experienced trauma and struggle with anorexia or other eating problems. Often bright, straight-A students or CEOs, they navigate the unemotional world of academics or computers brilliantly. Perceiving and managing their feelings, however, is more difficult. While they unconsciously or consciously deny that something is wrong, their shrinking bodies tell the truth: their buried emotions are literally eating away at them.

While anorexia and other eating disorders are complex disorders with biological, psychological, and social components, studies suggest that in people who have anorexia, the link between being able to understand and express their feelings is broken, and the damage is often caused by emotional, physical, or sexual trauma.

For example, some survivors of sexual abuse keep the abuse to themselves at the time of the incident, thereby not having the opportunity to process their initial reactions with trusted others. Or they may have extreme difficulty understanding and integrating the complexity of what happened to them. For example, if, as a child, a woman was abused by a beloved uncle, she may have felt both love and betrayal and doesn't know how to reconcile those two dissimilar emotions. Without understanding, there are no words. Unfortunately, that broken link between feelings and words can't fix itself.

Survivors may also cut themselves off from all feelings. In some abuse situations, they may dissociate. That coping style may pop up later when something else triggers the same feeling. For example, maybe a woman felt unsafe and violated by a teacher as a child. Later, when she feels her job is at risk and her boss can't be trusted, the same initial feeling may cause emotional turmoil. She couldn't talk about it then and can't talk about it now.

Again, not everyone with eating problems has been abused. What is common is that people who have difficulty expressing, understanding, and articulating their feelings, whether it's prompted by trauma or another deficit, often develop eating problems.

The good news is that those who have alexithymia can work through it. In fact, this is an essential part of the healing process. In counseling, men and women learn to connect the dots between how they feel and how those feelings affect their eating (starving, stuffing) and how to cope with those feelings. For example, they can learn that whenever they restrict their eating, they are feeling an "unacceptable" emotion, commonly anger. Making this connection in the moment can give them the opportunity to talk about their anger and deal with it in healthier ways rather than starving or overeating.

If this sounds like you, it's important to get good support and treatment. A qualified therapist can help you through the process and lead the way to healing.

The Healing Balm of Resilience

On September 11, 2001, the United States experienced a collective trauma: the bombing of the World Trade Center. As a nation, America was psychologically shattered. But the nation, and the survivors themselves, went on. We plumbed—and perhaps surprised ourselves with—the depths of our resilience.

Resilience is the process of bouncing back from adversity, trauma, or tragedy. The journey to resilience includes perceiving, accepting, and talking about distressing emotions—the very essence of emotional intelligence.

In fact, EI and resilience may have a direct link. In a recent study, French and Australian researchers had 414 people complete a scientific questionnaire that measures EI. Based on their scores, the participants were divided into three categories—vulnerable, average, and resilient—and the scores were calculated for six subscales: emotional self-awareness and emotional awareness of others, both of which concern perceiving and understanding your own and others' feelings; emotional expression, which focuses on effectively expressing your emotions; emotional self-control, which is the capacity to control your own intense feelings; emotional management of self and emotional management of others, both of which concern managing your own and others' emotions.

Emotional self-awareness, emotional expression, emotional self-control, and particularly emotional self-management appeared central to bouncing back after negative events, the researchers found.[13]

You might be wondering if you can develop these qualities. The answer is yes. And the key is to stand your ground emotionally. An acquaintance in a twelve-step program often quotes its various slogans. One of her favorites is: "Fear can mean F**k Everything And Run, or Face Everything And Recover."

To develop resilience requires that you face everything; and if you do, even imperfectly, you can recover. As a therapist, I've witnessed extraordinary resiliencey with very difficult (sometimes horrific) examples of trauma. It's possible to be happy and healthy no matter what you've experienced. Many of my clients who have experienced trauma or loss report positive changes after understanding the impact of their trauma. They report more satisfying relationships, a greater sense of strength even while feeling vulnerable, an increased sense of self-worth, and a more developed spirituality. Or they rethink what is truly important to them and come to appreciate what they value most in life.

To build your resilience, you'll need relationships rooted in love and trust, social support, a positive view of yourself, the ability to recognize your strengths, and a genuine belief that good things will happen in your life. It's easier to access these things when you can regulate your emotions. To regulate them, you need to build your emotional intelligence. And to do that, it's helpful to muster up your courage and talk about the situation or event that has left you voiceless, with food as your only source of comfort.

FOUR WAYS TO BOOST YOUR EATING RESILIENCE

Changing your eating habits isn't easy, which is why many of my clients have tried more than once. So I am always inspired when clients who have slipped off their healthy eating plans tell me, "I'm willing to give it another shot." The tips below can help you get some of their inspiring ability to bounce back.

1. *Cover the basics.* With adequate sleep, physical activity, and healthy food, you can better cope with the challenges that come your way—without overeating. *Tip:* Commit to getting seven to nine hours of sleep a night. Once you've met that goal, commit to moving your body for thirty minutes, three times a week.

2. *Embrace slips as teachable moments.* My most resilient clients view every slip as an opportunity to learn ways to manage that scenario more effectively next time. *Tip:* If you should happen to slip, ask yourself, "What did I learn?"

3. *Open your mind.* Instead of doing what *doesn't* work over and over again, my resilient clients say, "This just isn't working. I have to try something new." *Tip:* Try a tool from this book that isn't already in your repertoire of skills.

4. *Seek social support.* My most resilient clients reach out for support when they need it. While they may not find it easy to ask for help, they do it because they know it works. *Tip:* Talk with a support group, friend, coworker, or therapist—anyone who is willing to listen.

KRISTINE'S STORY

Because research shows a high correlation between eating problems and sexual abuse, I work with many survivors, and many have eating disorders. Often their compulsive eating is a visible sign that their bodies have become battlefields. While some open up to me about the abuse or violence right away, others need time to develop trust and feel safe.

Kristine, a thirty-seven-year-old occupational therapist, needed that time. A lovely, intelligent woman, engaging and funny, she was also a closet eater, eating like a "good girl" in public but overeating at home. Forty pounds overweight, she wrote "body image" and "overeating" on her intake sheet. But she was also concerned about her relationships and her difficulty with dating. Although Kristine alluded to an incident with a babysitter, which occurred when she was around seven years old, she dodged my gentle questions about it, and I didn't press.

After a few months of sessions, she began dating a man she'd met at work. As the relationship progressed, Kristine wanted to express her feelings physically, but in an intimate moment she suddenly recoiled.

"It was the way he held my arm down against the bed," she said. "Until that moment I was totally into it. But that slight action—I panicked and pulled away. It was automatic. The moment was ruined. Things between us are weird now. I feel permanently damaged. I can never have a normal relationship." Time and again we returned to this underlying sense of herself.

In her pain, she was ready to talk about the abuse. After the story tumbled out, I offered her a tissue and soft words of comfort.

"There's no such thing as 'permanently damaged,'" I said. "The trauma you experienced affects how you view yourself and engage in the world. Sometimes it makes you shut down. Sometimes it makes you distrustful. It has definitely affected your eating. But it does not define who you are. And you *can* have a normal, healthy relationship that includes physical intimacy. It will take time and courage, but we've got plenty of time, and I sense that you have the courage."

I was right. After several months, she began to turn a corner in regards to her eating and dating. But first, she had to get a clear sense of how the past was affecting her present.

Like Kristine, many of the trauma survivors I work with consciously or unconsciously blame themselves for the abuse. Sometimes they see it as the underlying reason they feel unlovable or struggle in their relationships. Survivors of any type of abuse benefit from learning to perceive and accept their feelings and give them voice. When they talk about their abuse—explain how it shaped their identities, life choices, attitudes about food—the feelings it engenders are less likely to surface in moments of intimacy or shape their eating.

Perhaps the hardest thing for a survivor of abuse to believe is that what happened—this horrifying, life-changing event—is, in some ways, like a scar on your knee. You know where it came from and how it got there. You have a story to tell about it. Sometimes things happen that trigger your memory of how it got there.

I'm not equating sexual abuse to a scarred knee. I'm telling you something about the process of healing. A scar is your skin's way of repairing itself from injury; think too of the scar on a woman's chest left by the mastectomy that saved her life.

Scars on souls form for the same reason: they are signs of healing. But scars can heal in healthy or unhealthy ways. To help a scar to the soul heal in a healthy way, it sometimes takes looking at it without turning away. Then you must tell the story of how it came to be there and deal with the feelings your story elicits in healing ways. If you do this, the scar will heal well. You will always carry it, but it will no longer be the only thing you see.

Resilience Has a Voice

How does expressing feelings and using emotional intelligence help a person recover from trauma? Let me answer with a true and very personal story.

Several years ago, in a spontaneous moment, I decided to elope to Italy. I packed an incredible gown, picked a spot in Venice, and lined up housing with extended family members who own a vineyard. We flew into Rome, picked up our rental car and, just outside the city, pulled over at a rest stop to use the restroom. We locked the car and were gone for only a moment.

When we returned, the car was empty. The robbers had stuck a screwdriver in the trunk lock and broken it open. Wedding dress and veil, passports, cameras, luggage—all were stolen in broad daylight.

I remember scanning the parking lot, which was filled with tractor-trailers and people who, to my traumatized mind, seemed to be lurking. Whoever made off with our property was likely watching my reaction to the theft. To make a long story short, it was not quite the wedding I had planned and my sense of safety and security evaporated. I'm an experienced traveler. This spot had appeared safe to me.

Over the years, I've listened to myself tell the story over and over again. Although the ending never changes—I still get robbed—the way I tell the story has evolved over the years. When I first returned from the trip, the tale was imbued with my fear and sense of violation—there was someone in the world who had my clothing and pictures of me! Then, it turned to a tale of woe—the wedding that I had so rapturously envisioned didn't happen.

But somewhere along the line, it has turned into a tale of resilience. I focus on how we coped with losing our passports and survived for two weeks without any clothes and barely a dime between us.

My point is that as my feelings about the robbery changed, so did my story. But it was the fact that I *told* the story—expressed the fear, sense of violation, sadness, and anger—that helped me heal.

Of course, not all traumas eventually end well and can transform into a tale of resilience. But what is important is *telling* your story, whether to a friend or a counselor. Had I kept mine to myself, locked it away in my heart, I'm not sure it would have had the opportunity to transform in the way it did. Healing comes from expressing and understanding the way we feel—the essence of emotional intelligence.

REBECCA'S STORY

Flying home from a business conference, flipping through a women's magazine, Rebecca stumbled on an article on the factors that affect a woman's body image. In the story, I was quoted as saying that trauma is one of those factors.

"My heart stopped. I started to cry; my entire face was wet with tears," the forty-year-old computer analyst told me at our first meeting. "It was the first time I had connected my weight with something that had happened to me a long time ago. I called your office for an appointment as soon as I got home."

Then, she haltingly revealed her story, untold for nearly two decades.

In college, on a holiday with her roommates, Rebecca had been accosted in the hallway of her hotel. Her assailant was a boy in her class she knew only by his first name. Silent, he had pinned her against the wall, covered her mouth with his hand, and fondled her. She was paralyzed with fear—would he rape her? Drag her into his room and kill her?

Her assailant had, by force, taken from Rebecca two vital qualities essential to one's well-being: the abilities to feel safe and to trust. That her friends neither understood nor validated the intensity of her fear and anger increased her feelings of isolation.

When she saw her assailant in class the following week, he didn't even look at her.

"It was like nothing happened," she said. "This made me feel crazy. I started second-guessing myself—did it really happen, or did I make it up? Also, he looked 'normal'—a nice guy in a baseball cap who spoke politely in class. Now, it's like there's no way to tell the dangerous men from the nice ones."

Rebecca became hypervigilant, constantly scanning her environment for danger. When she walked into a room, she examined the men closely. If one looked even a little unsavory, she'd leave. A relationship, or even a casual date, was out of the question.

Unable to cope with her overwhelming feelings of fear, anger, and isolation, she smothered them with food. Of average weight at the time of the assault, she gained fifty pounds in the years following. Insomnia became a problem. Numbed by high-fat, high-sugar foods like cookie dough and milk shakes, she'd fall into a "food coma," which allowed her to sleep.

Almost twenty years later, Rebecca remained torn between her need to feel safe and her sense of loneliness. My job was to help her discover that deep down she held on to her extra weight as protection. It formed a wall around her. Men were less likely to approach or harm her.

Before we tackled Rebecca's relationship issues, we needed to connect her eating and her feelings. After the assault, she'd linked eating high-fat, high-sugar comfort foods with relief from painful feelings, and that connection had to be broken.

To help Rebecca begin to embrace those painful emotions (the E in the EAT method), I asked her to list on paper her feelings about the assault. Because she'd repressed them for almost twenty years, bringing them to the surface could immediately create a tsunami of emotion that would engulf her.

Next, I asked her to read what she'd written to me. With time, she learned to talk about those feelings without writing them out first. In other words, she was able to integrate the assault into her experience.

Accepting her feelings (A) was more difficult. Rebecca had been using food to numb out for almost twenty years, and it didn't stop overnight. At times, she'd rationalize her binges. For a time she stopped soothing her feelings with food, but she began drinking wine instead. She stopped when she realized that she'd simply substituted one numbing agent for another. Keeping a food diary helped her be honest about her overeating and binges, and breathing exercises helped her sit with the anger and fear.

We also worked on finding new ways to manage her feelings (T). Rebecca discovered that mindless activities—flipping through a magazine, knitting, zoning out in front of the TV—calmed her the most. Mild

▶

exercise—a brisk walk in a nearby park, for example—helped her drift off to sleep without the self-medication of fat and sugar.

Rebuilding her sense of safety and trust—the primary building blocks of any intimate relationship—took time. Rebecca had to trust that she could not only protect herself physically (by meeting her date at the restaurant instead of having him pick her up, for example) without isolating herself, but that she could trust her intuition to tell her if she could feel truly safe with a man over time.

I admired Rebecca's courage in finally confronting her trauma. It would have been easier to close the magazine and remain on her self-sabotaging path. But her longing for love and connection outweighed her fear. At the moment when she felt the most helpless and vulnerable—sobbing over a magazine article on a plane—she chose to live. She is now dating—and enjoying it.

Rebecca refused to allow a traumatic experience to define who she is and affect her health and emotional well-being. You can do it too, if you're willing to examine rather than erase the past. The journey to reclaiming your past can be the scariest—and most rewarding—of your life.

Coping with Trauma

The EAT method can help you work through trauma and untangle its hold on your eating. It worked for Amy, who was in university when she came to me for help with her compulsive eating.

Amy grew up poor on a family farm. She and her eight brothers and sisters worked long and hard. One of Amy's many chores was to rise before dawn to feed the cows. During the punishing winters, her hands froze to the metal pail, leaving them raw and bleeding. Her stomach didn't fare much better. In such a large, poor family, barely hanging on to its farm, there was rarely enough food.

Amy's mother served breakfast after morning chores. Amy and her siblings would literally elbow each other out of the way to get at the food. When
Amy was lucky enough to get breakfast—and she wasn't always lucky—she
swallowed without chewing. Lunch and dinner brought the same desperate
wrestling matches at the table. She also stole food from friends' houses or,
when she could, hoarded food in a dresser drawer.

With the EAT method, Amy was able to move past her early feelings of
deprivation and stop overeating in the present.

E: Identify

If you are having an extreme reaction, identify whether your feelings are
blocked (numb, disconnected), blurred (confused, triggering past feelings in
the present), or ballooned (exaggerated) by taking the quiz (on page 198). In
Amy's case, her trigger was the buffet-style canteen at college. For Amy, it
created blurred and ballooned feelings at the same time. The unlimited food
and many choices triggered the little girl inside, who'd had to fight for and
hoard food to get enough (blurring). Each time she entered the canteen Amy
experienced panic, as if she should eat as much as possible before it disap-
peared (ballooning).

Once she perceived that the abundance she saw triggered the panic, Amy
decided to eat at the canteen at the same times each day, which helped to
defuse the panic. To a survivor of trauma, structure and routine can be very
calming. So, if this sounds like you, first identify how your feelings may be
skewed.

A: Understand What's Happened

Honor the fact that your responses to your distorted feelings helped you cope
with the trauma. But today that coping style has become the problem. Amy
needed to appreciate that anyone as constantly hungry as she had been as a
child would, as an adult, eat frantically in the presence of seemingly unlimited amounts of food. Grabbing and eating as much as possible when she
had the opportunity served her well at one juncture in her life. At this point,
however, food was always available. She was safe and okay. It was her coping
response that was outdated, and it was time to change it. My validation of
Amy's eating behavior helped her accept it and get ready to move on from it.

If this sounds like you, reestablish a sense of safety. Remind yourself that you're in a different situation. Create actual safety if you need to—in Amy's case having a friend go with her to meals helped increase in her a feeling of safety that she wouldn't lose control. Then mentally return to the present and center yourself with Q-TIPP and mindful meditation.

T: Talk About It

Talking can help you get your feelings back in check and realign your skewed feelings. You may want to test the waters by writing in your journal (it's like talking to yourself). Discuss how your feelings might be blocked, blurred, or ballooned. Or talk to someone close to you or a counselor. You might also open up to a trusted friend or family member. Talking can help put your feelings back into perspective, help you regain trust in them, and connect your trauma, your feelings, and your eating.

Amy didn't want to talk about her past with her friends. She experimented with another outlet for self-expression: journaling. As she wrote about her childhood hunger, she understood that now, as an adult, she was capable of taking care of herself and making sure she had enough to eat.

Healing from trauma was difficult for Amy, and it may be difficult for you. This chapter may help you connect the dots between your experiences, emotions, and eating. But if you need more help (and many people do), please schedule an appointment with a therapist who specializes in treating trauma and/or eating issues.

The Last Bite

If you have experienced a trauma or situation that greatly affected your feelings, I hope you have gained a sense of support and hope from this chapter. Challenging experiences can alter and skew your emotions, making them murky and unclear. This is normal. Yet these experiences also give you an opportunity to get to know yourself and your tremendous capacity for resiliencey and growth. Trauma doesn't have to define who you are or how you eat. You have the capacity to bounce back, to recover and thrive.

PART THREE

Tools for Success

Our feelings are our most genuine paths to knowledge.

—Audre Lorde

What a wonderful quote to begin this section! It's my hope that in part 3 you will begin to walk those paths—some pleasant, others challenging—and transform the theory of emotional intelligence into your reality. But before we dive into the tools, let's recap what you've learned so far.

In parts 1 and 2 we examined the theory of EI and how its four dimensions—the abilities to perceive, understand, use, and manage feelings—affect your relationship with food. If those abilities aren't where they need to be or you don't apply them to your eating, you'll undermine your power to pause, examine your foreground and background, and make those all-important insight-driven choices. Simply put, you'll continue to make the same emotion-driven decisions that lead to emotional eating, over-eating, and weight gain.

You've also "met" some of my clients, whose struggles to manage their emotions affected their eating decisions, their abilities to withstand a craving or bounce back from a slip or binge, and their weight. More often than not, those who fully embrace the EAT method lose weight and make peace with food. It's my hope that you found some of your story—and hope—in theirs.

Now, in part 3, you'll learn twenty-five tools to help you take a mindful pause and apply the EAT method in virtually any situation. The E tools help you identify exactly what you're feeling in the moment of decision, the A tools help you use your feelings to make insight-driven decisions, and the T tools give you specific ways to cope with your feelings so you don't automatically act on your impulse to eat. Together, the tools give you the skills you need to put the four dimensions of emotional intelligence into practice—anywhere, anytime.

Practice is the key word. Part 3 gives you the tools but, like muscles, they require frequent use. You'll find some tools more helpful than others, and that's okay. But do give each a try. You might also start an Eat.Q. notebook, so you can write out certain exercises or jot notes on each tool. (Some tools involve writing—nothing complicated—and it's nice to have your jottings in one place, the simpler to work, ponder, and peruse.)

The tools aren't foolproof; sometimes, in the eternal struggle between cheesecake and waistline, the cheesecake will win. It's impossible to manage every feeling or always make the "right" or healthy decision. What I can promise is that if you use the tools faithfully, you'll know yourself better and depend on food for comfort less and less often. You'll be able to perceive, predict, and prepare for feelings that drive you to food.

Let's get started! I hope you're ready to dive into simple yet practical exercises that will take your Eat.Q. to the next level.

9

E

Embracing Your Feelings, Learning to Reconnect

Let's not forget that the little emotions are the great captains
of our lives and we obey them without realizing it.

—Vincent Van Gogh

The E tools sharpen your ability to identify and verbalize your feelings and evaluate their effect on your behavior. In other words, they're the raw material of insight-driven decisions. They're also the foundation on which the A and T tools rest. To show you how vital they are to raising Eat.Q., here's a before-and-after scenario:

Before you learn and use the E tools:
I overate because I was angry at my partner.

After you learn and use the E tools:
*I was angry at my partner and wanted to eat, so I went for
a walk to cool off instead.*

See the difference? In the first example, your feelings overruled your decision. In the second, your awareness of your emotions changed your behavior.

The sooner you perceive, appraise, and express your feelings in the moment, the more likely you are to stick to your eating plan. Let's say you've just left a long, frustrating meeting. It's time for your mid-morning snack. You have a plastic bag of almonds from home, but you're craving cake. Armed with your E tools, you know that you're angry and frustrated. Using one or more of the following tools (you're bound to have a favorite or two) can help you short-circuit the anger, defuse the craving, and stick with your healthy snack. The tools in this section draw on mindfulness, emotional fluency (lots of word games!), and reading your body's cues to uncover what you're feeling. Every time you put one into practice, you boost your Eat.Q.

Tool 1: Build Your Emotional Vocabulary

Remember that old children's song that begins, "When you're happy and you know it, clap your hands"? In this exercise, you'll raise your ability to differentiate between "shades" of the same emotion. It's wonderful if you're angry and you know it. Even better, however, is to know that you're irritated or resentful—subtle variations of anger. Searching for exactly the right word to name your feeling affords you a pause, which strengthens impulse control and empowers you to cope with that feeling in a positive way.

Verbalizing sadness and anger makes these powerful emotions less intense, and putting negative feelings into words activates a part of the brain responsible for impulse control, according to a study conducted at the University of California, Los Angeles.[1] In this study, thirty people were shown pictures of faces expressing strong emotions. As the researchers administered brain scans, the volunteers were asked to categorize the feelings in words like "sad" or "angry," or choose between two gender-specific names, such as "Sally" or "Harry," that matched the face.

Attaching a word like "angry" to an angry-looking face reduced the response in the amygdala, the part of the brain that deals with fear, panic, and other strong emotions, the researchers found.

However, when the volunteers labeled the feeling, another region of their brains became *more* active: the right ventrolateral prefrontal cortex. Research has linked this region with thinking in words about emotional experiences, processing emotions, and inhibiting behavior.[2]

What does all this mean to you? A lot, if you're a stress or emotional eater. It's a big deal to know what you feel so well that you can describe it in one precise word. That skill helps you gain greater insight into what your emotions want you to do (eat!) and strips them of much of their power. Building your feelings vocabulary may strengthen your impulse control, enabling you to withstand cravings or skip extra helpings.

But the ability to name your feelings isn't always easy. First, we're used to using generic words to describe our feelings. How many times have you been asked how you feel and responded with "okay" or "fine"? If you're in the habit of giving such rote, unspecific responses to others, you may talk to yourself using the same bland, unemotional vocabulary.

Moreover, if you grew up in a family that didn't acknowledge or talk about emotions, or you were shushed or made fun of for expressing your feelings, you are not likely to have much experience attaching feeling words to your experiences. What would it have been like if, as a child, when you fell down and skinned your knee, your mother or other caregiver scooped you up and said, "Oh, sweetie, you must feel scared and hurt." Such empathy and modeling of feelings strengthens the cognitive connections between the feeling and the word.

Finally, emotions are complex, fleeting, and often conflicting. For example, in the aftermath of a breakup, it isn't easy finding the right word to express simultaneously loving and hating your ex. (It can be enough to say that you feel both love and hate, which feels confusing and painful.) The complexity of trying to capture fleeting or extreme feelings may prevent us from even trying.

However, it's possible to become downright eloquent in describing how you feel, even if you've had trouble with it in the past. I've had clients who used to shrug helplessly or struggle for words when I asked them to describe, in detail, what they were feeling. But as they practiced the following exercise, they began to name their feelings as if they'd been doing it all their lives.

You can do this too. The better you become at labeling what you feel in the moment—frustrated, lonely, listless, irritated, etc.—the less likely you are to impulsively reach for food to make the confusion go away. A "wheel of emotions" was developed by preeminent psychologist Robert Plutchik thirty years ago. Since then, many other feelings wheels have been created. They show that, like colors, primary emotions can mix with one another to form different emotions.

Here's an example of a feelings wheel that I've created.

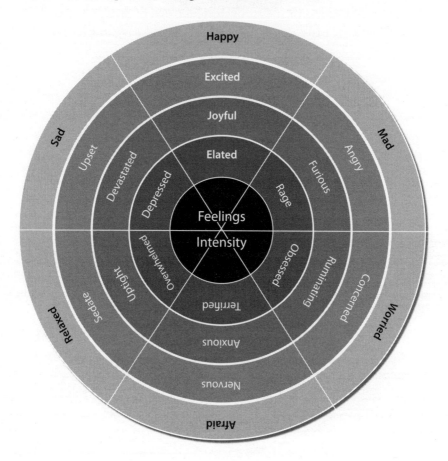

Now, it's time to create your own, using the blank feelings wheel on the next page. Doing this exercise can help you push beyond generic responses such as "fine" or "okay." Opposite is a blank feelings wheel I've designed just for this exercise; it's designed to be photocopied.

EXERCISE

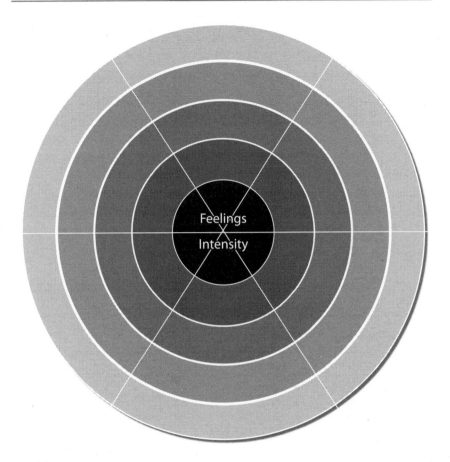

STEP 1

On the outer rim of the wheel, write in the primary emotion you tend to feel most often (*sad, glad, mad,* and so forth).

In the spaces toward the wheel of the circle, write in more descriptive and specific words (*depressed, irritated, joyful*).

If you feel empty, bored, or flat, write that down. They're emotions, too.

If you don't know how you feel, that's okay. Just acknowledge that and repeat the exercise in an hour. You might also try to fill in the gap later.

In the beginning, you may process feelings more clearly after they've passed.

Keep your completed wheel with you, perhaps in your Eat.Q. notebook. Then, for the next two days, once an hour, stop what you're doing and name an emotion you have experienced in the past ten minutes.

As your ability to process and name your feelings improves, keep in touch with your feelings and begin a new wheel. (Make a stack of copies, so you'll always have a fresh one on hand.)

STEP 2

Just as we have "shades" of feelings, we have "shades" of hunger, as well as many words to describe our emotional experiences of eating. Step 2 is designed to increase your emotional vocabulary related to food and eating.

Repeat step 1, adding a word to describe any desire or urge to eat you experienced in the past ten minutes. Here are a few words to get you thinking:

- full
- stuffed
- satisfied
- ravenous
- starving
- craving
- obsessing
- guilt
- anticipation

I recommend that you practice this part of the exercise at least twice a day, and more often if you wish. As measuring your food helps you be conscious of portion control, naming your feelings keeps you aware of the power they wield over your eating decisions.

Tool 2: Words That Make You Go "Mmm"

Politicians and preachers know the power of words. So do food marketers, who use words like *silky* or *succulent* or *home-style* or *farm-fresh* strategically to evoke specific emotions—pleasure, comfort, nostalgia, purity.

Such emotion-laden words can hit us in the gut and shape our food decisions. We respond automatically, often leagues below our emotional radar. A study conducted by Brian Wansink and colleagues found that sales increased 27 percent based on the words used to describe a menu item—for example, "New York–Style Cheesecake with Godiva Chocolate Sauce" versus "cheesecake." The former sounds much tastier, doesn't it? More indulgent? Yet they're both just cheesecake.[3]

In the same way words can draw you into eating, they can also sabotage you. In my work, I've found that the word *diet* triggers deep emotions. While a few people feel motivated when they hear it, most experience visceral feelings of failure and fear.

How about you? Close your eyes. Repeat the word to yourself aloud (or silently).

Diet.

Diet.

Diet.

What did you feel in your body as you said this word? Did your heart sink or your stomach knot up? Did you clench your jaw or slump in your seat just a bit? Did saying it make you feel angry, helpless, or powerless?

I often do the following two exercises with my clients. In both, we'll first use IQ to explore what we know intellectually about the words. Then we'll tap into Eat.Q. to reveal the *feelings* the words evoke—feelings that can lead to emotion-driven decisions. You'll need a pen and your Eat.Q. notebook.

Knowing Versus Feeling

1. Divide a page in your Eat.Q. notebook into three vertical columns (either fold it in thirds or draw straight lines down the length of the paper).

2. Label the first column "Words." On the next lines, write these six items, one to a line:

   - Health

   - Calorie

   - Comfort food

   - Thin

   - Dine

   - Overeat

3. Label the second column "Definitions" and the third "Emotions."

4. In the second column, write the literal definition of each item. Use a dictionary if you'd like, but try to define it in your own words. (You're forcing your brain to *think* about the literal meaning of each word.)

5. In the third column, list the emotions attached to each item. Don't censor yourself, just free-associate, scribbling whatever words or phrases come to mind. Be aware, too, of words that elicit positive emotional responses. For example, when I say the phrase "mindful eating," people tend to nod and smile. Do any of the emotional words make you nod or smile—*low-sugar,* perhaps, or *whole grain*? They're important to notice; you can home in on them as you decide what to eat.

6. Compare the definition with the emotion. As an example, let's consider the word *calorie*. Intellectually, you may know a calorie is a unit of heat. But what does the word *calorie* mean to you emotionally?

One of my clients wrote:

> Fear
>
> Anger
>
> Stupid
>
> Energy
>
> Restriction
>
> Salads [this particular client loathed salads]

Armed with your list of emotion-triggering words, sort them into two categories: those that motivate you and those that evoke negative feelings. In the example above, *energy* is an example of one word that could be motivating.

When you know which words trigger those negative emotions that lurk below the surface of your consciousness, you'll likely make decisions that are driven by insight rather than emotion. Let's say you're at a restaurant that, by law, must post nutrition information for its menu items. On the menu, you read the word "calories." You think, *Ugh. Diet food.* Annoyed (but not aware of that annoyance), you turn away and impulsively order what you want.

Let's replay that scene, this time using Eat.Q.

Ugh. Diet food. I admit it. The word calorie *annoys me. I hate considering calories when I'm hungry or out to dinner. But I also don't want a mere word to hold such power over me. I can make a healthy choice.*

EXERCISE

Deconstructing a Menu

1. The next time you're at a restaurant, analyze the name of each entrée on the menu and the words used to describe it.

2. Next, read the descriptions of each entrée. Make a mental note of enticing words, such as "tender," "flaky," "sizzling," "vine-ripened," and so forth.

3. Finally, delete every descriptive word, stripping the description to its basic meaning. You may have questions to ask your server, too. For example, this is what the menu says: "Home-Style Sicilian Veal Parmesan. A plump, deep-fried veal patty, lightly breaded, topped with a sauce of vine-ripened tomatoes and smothered in mozzarella." And this is what it actually is: a fried, breaded, processed-veal patty topped with tomato sauce (are the tomatoes literally vine-ripened— straight from a local farm—or are you getting sauce from a jar?) and mozzarella cheese. Also, what makes it "home-style"—or "Sicilian," for that matter?

4. Ponder how much the names and descriptions of the entrées pull you in emotionally. Which words make your mouth water? Did decoding the descriptions dampen your ardor? Is the food that makes your mouth water really worth eating? If so, why?

Make a habit of deconstructing entrée names and descriptions each time you eat out. It's a great way to insert a mindful pause into a situation ripe for an emotion-driven decision.

Tool 3: Be Here

On Facebook, a friend recently posted that she'd mistakenly started to apply toothpaste (!) to her face. She'd thought it was her prescription skin cream—also in a tube—and didn't notice until she tuned in to the gritty texture and the overpowering odor of mint.

We all act on autopilot—perhaps in the morning, before coffee, or while driving. That *zoning out* we do, followed by an abrupt *tuning in*? That happens with eating, too. You know what I mean if you've ever munched from a bag of crisps while reading a novel or watching a movie, and then suddenly you tuned in and realized that you've eaten three-quarters of the bag.

If that sounds like you, the technique of mindfulness will be wonderfully helpful. This exercise was inspired by a monk I "met" in Kyoto, Japan. Visiting the Ryōan-ji temple, known for its abstract rock garden, you'd think I'd be absorbed in the beauty around me, but no. I had my nose buried in my tourist's guidebook. Where to go next? Another temple? Back to the hotel?

The monk—who I'd not even noticed—must have seen my distraction, because he drew near and tapped me on the arm. *"Be here,"* he whispered in a calm, kind voice.

Jolted back into the moment, I simply stared at his serene countenance. But his simple two-word instruction has stayed with me, a shorthand reminder to bring myself and others back to the moment—to change from zoned out to tuned in. If you need a visual, imagine someone whispering to you, trying to get your attention, saying, "Hey. Over here. *Look*." That's mindfulness. The following tool is often one of the first techniques I teach my clients before I venture into the specifics of changing their eating habits.

EXERCISE

Silently or aloud, repeat the phrase "Be here" each time you eat, before you take even one bite. If you're trying to decide on a snack, say, "Be here," and *then* decide.

Also, repeat it every time you notice that you've zoned out, to bring yourself back to what you're feeling at that moment.

When you notice yourself thinking of a hundred different things at once . . . *Be here.*

If you're texting, talking, and barking out orders to your kids at the same time . . . *Be here.*

If you're feeling frantic and overwhelmed . . . *Be here.*

Also, to help you begin the process, here's a simple trick that can help you practice:

Halt. Slow down. Give yourself one minute to check in—yes, one minute is all you need.

Engage in the present moment. Focus on what is going on *right now.*

Research and gather data on your foreground and background (see chapter 6). Research is objective data—no judgment attached. Focus on your senses and what your body is telling you about how you feel.

Embrace the emotion. Welcome in whatever you're feeling right now—good feelings, bad feelings, whatever they may be.

Once you identify the feeling, you can use this critical information in your decision-making process. Do you feel anger or stress, and feel the urge to overeat to quell that feeling? Do you feel happy and calm and want to prolong that feeling of well-being with food?

Practice this exercise a few times, and you'll start to instantly recognize when you zone out and know how to bring yourself back into the moment, so you can make smarter decisions. I recall one client telling me about sitting in a restaurant, mindlessly picking at the rolls in the bread basket. She silently whispered to herself, "*Be here*," and in a minute or so tuned in to the fact that she was anxious, not hungry. She asked the server to remove the basket, and that was that.

To dig deeper into the specific skill of mindful eating, consider cooking more. With its chopping and peeling, mixing and blending, the bouquet of aromas and beautiful colors, it's an activity exquisitely suited to mindfulness. As you peel and slice cucumbers and bell peppers and carrots for your salad, be there. When you mix your vinaigrette, be there. Focus on the fragrance of fresh basil, the sharp sweet smell of balsamic vinegar, the sound of your knife on your chopping board. Even if you cook twice a week, in a mindful way, you'll reap some benefits. Research shows that people who cook more lose more weight.

Finally, try to live each day in this state of heightened awareness. When you walk, breathe in the scent of rain on earth (or concrete), tune in to the heat of the sun on your head, watch your feet scuffle through leaves and enjoy the crunch underfoot. When you encounter people, focus on their body language—their gestures, the pitch of their voices. Vacuum the carpet mindfully; shower mindfully. Focus your mind, savor the *here*, and accept what you feel. Experience how much richer life is inside the shimmering bubble of *now*.

Tool 4: Firm Your Muscles, Firm Your Resolve

I am a healthy eater.
I absolutely will not have another bite!
Many of my clients use positive thinking to stick to their eating plans, but it doesn't work all the time. When thinking positive isn't doing the trick, add another component: muscle.

In one of a series of studies, researchers in Singapore found that tightening your muscles—an action that frequently accompanies mental resolve—can help you summon the resolve you need to make better food choices.[4] This finding is one of many in a relatively new branch of psychology known as *embodied cognition,* which posits that your brain looks to your face and body to understand how you feel. In other words, the instant you make up your mind, declaring "This is it!" your muscles, reflecting that thought, contract naturally. You might grimace, grit your teeth, or clench your fist.

Studies of embodied cognition have elicited some truly fascinating findings. For example, in a study led by Yale psychologist John Bargh, people holding warm cups of coffee, rather than cold cups, were more inclined to judge a research associate as trustworthy after only a short elevator ride together. Similarly, at the University of Toronto people were asked to remember a time when they were either socially accepted or snubbed. Those who recalled warm welcomes judged the room to be, on average, five degrees warmer than those who remembered rejection—the equivalent of a chilly reception.[5] Thus, your bodily sensations can play a significant role in shaping how you feel and think.

When your mind and body are working in tandem, it's easier to connect with your emotions. For example, the cognitive aspects of anger (knowing you're angry) are tied to the physical aspects of anger (feeling it in your body—a knotted stomach, clenched fists, shallow breathing). Similarly, feelings of sadness can lead to crying or sobbing, a sensation experienced in the body. Significantly, those who can't cry after a trauma, such as the loss of a loved one, often report feeling frustrated and emotionally confused.

Many people unknowingly create a split between body and mind. You've experienced this split if you've ever smiled and nodded as your boss was talking, while thinking silently, *I can't stand this woman.* Or, for that matter, if you've ever thought *Stop eating! Now!* as your hand continued to move from the bag of crisps to your mouth.

In the Singapore study, the researchers divided sixty-six people, whom they had recruited at a university campus snack bar, into two groups. Both groups were given a pen and different sets of instructions. The first group was told to grasp the pen (which firmed the muscles in their fingers). The second group was instructed to simply hold the pen (no muscle firming involved).

Then, as the subjects ordered food at the same campus snack bar, the researchers evaluated their choices. Those who grasped the pen reportedly had more willpower. They also chose healthier options. The muscles' actions appear to mirror the mind's wishes, the study suggests. It's worth noting, however, that even in the pen-grasping group, only those who *wanted* to exert self-control over their food choices did so.

The following exercise is not a magic bullet, but it can be a very helpful tool.

EXERCISE

As tools go, this one is elegantly simple. The next time you struggle with saying no to food, clench your fists or tighten your calf muscles or biceps as you say, silently or aloud, "No." Repeat this several times, focusing on how it feels when your mind joins forces with your muscles.

Or simply grasp a pen, as the volunteers in the study did. As you clench it, think *No!* to let your body know you mean business.

Tool 5: Emotional Status Updates

How often do you check your e-mail, Facebook or Twitter? Once a week, once a day, once a minute? Those instant updates can keep you on top of the news—you know what's happening, as it's happening, anywhere in the world and can stay in constant touch with friends and family. The downside, however, is that you can become so immersed in what is happening "out there" that you forget to stay tuned in to what's making headlines in your inner world. Checking your in-box can be a distraction from, or even an escape from, what you're feeling inside. The solution is to continually "refresh" your emotional status.

Your emotions are constantly changing from hour to hour, minute to minute. Once you understand how mobile your feelings are—how quickly they can change—it's easier to stay one step ahead of emotional eating. Living at warp speed can cut you off from your emotions and from true, belly-rumbling hunger. I have lots of super-busy mums, CEOs, and graduate students as clients, and they tell me that they aren't hungry during the day but then binge at night. It's not that they aren't hungry; they are too busy to notice they're hungry. They're caught in a whirlwind of the external rather than the internal world.

That doesn't have to happen to you. For example, if you notice the first signs of stress—low energy, tense muscles, a pounding headache—you can anticipate that chocolate will be calling your name any minute now. At that point, you still have time to push PAUSE and short-circuit that craving.

It takes mere seconds to update yourself; do it at least once a day (although you can do it as often as you wish). Set a regular time to update your emotional status. You can "refresh" every fifteen minutes, once an hour, or before routine tasks, such as sending an e-mail or making a phone call. You can do a general update or monitor a particular feeling, such as stress or anxiety. Then record your updates in your Eat.Q. notebook.

EXERCISE

1. Close your eyes and for several moments do focused breathing (chapter 2) to clear your mind and turn inward.

2. When you feel calm, gently ask yourself what else you're feeling in that moment. If you aren't sure, check your body language for clues. Are your shoulders tense, or are you jiggling your foot? (You may feel stressed.) Are you slumped over your desk or fiddling with a paper clip? (Perhaps you're bored or blue.) Are you breathing shallowly? (That suggests anxiety.)

If you have trouble with this exercise, ask yourself what you're feeling in the moment, then imagine your response as a newspaper headline: short and to the point. You might focus on something more specific, such as "My body is feeling . . ." or "How hungry am I at this moment?"

After a few days of updates, you may begin to notice ebbs and flows in your moods. Can you discern any patterns? If so, begin to anticipate and plan for those moods. If you make the clearest decisions in the morning, pack your lunch first thing in the morning. If you're typically in meltdown by the end of the day, snack in the mid-afternoon to short-circuit before-dinner cravings.

Tool 6: Rating *Want to Eat* Versus *Need to Eat*

I love the book *Intuitive Eating* by Evelyn Tribole and Elyse Resch so much that I keep several copies on the bookshelf in my office to lend to clients. First published in 1995 and now in its third edition, its message was (and remains) revolutionary: eat when you're hungry, and stop when you're full. In other words, rely on your body's internal cues to tell you when to stop and start eating. Hunger, the body's physical need for food signaled by a growling belly, is a basic internal cue. Other cues are more subtle and include a headache, low energy, or feeling grumpy or jittery.

Most of the time, however, we eat in response to external cues—TV commercials of juicy burgers, muffins sitting on the kitchen counter, a bag of crisps left on the coffee table. We respond to *appetite*—the *want to eat*—rather than hunger—the *need to eat*.[6] This is the reason we walk into the supermarket intending to buy milk, and walk out with a box of snack cakes that were on sale. There is an entire psychology behind impulse buying. It turns out that even if we don't think we are susceptible to impulse buying, we are!

Research conducted at Cornell University demonstrates the power of external cues, how they subtly—and often unconsciously—influence our eating decisions. In this study, researchers randomly assigned 122 people to one of two groups. Those in the first group were given "meal cues"—they were served a meal (quesadillas and chicken wings) at a table on real plates, with glasses, silverware, and cloth napkins. Those in the other group received "snack cues"—they were served the same items on paper plates and with paper napkins. They were given no utensils, drank from plastic cups, and ate standing up.

Participants given meal cues ate 28 percent more calories than participants in the snack-cue group (416 versus 532 calories on average), the study found. (The findings corroborated previous research that has shown that people tend to eat more at meals than at snack times.) The take-home message is that more often than we know or care to admit we respond to our background without zeroing in on our foreground (chapter 6).

This finding suggests that to increase your awareness of what and how much you eat, put your trust not in external cues—which can and often are manipulative—but in your internal cues of hunger and satiety—which are less likely to steer you wrong.[7] Once you've raised your Eat.Q. enough to identify the external cues that push your EAT! button, you can keep an eye out and prepare for them.

Typically, counselors and psychologists teach their clients to rate their hunger and fullness on a scale from one to ten before they take even one bite of food. However, you may miss the mark if you've learned to equate fullness with a stuffed belly, which suggests overeating. The goal is not to be *full* but to experience an absence of hunger and a feeling of satisfaction. There's a big difference! That's why I recommend that you learn to discern between emotional and physical hunger—*want to eat* versus *need to eat*. The *want* rating in the following exercise reveals the level of your desire for a particular food or the next bite. This is the emotional scale tapping into the search for pleasure or hedonistic desires. The *need* rating reveals your level of true physical hunger.

EXERCISE

Before each item you eat—whether meal, snack, or even a single nibble—ask yourself two brief questions. They'll train your mind to pause and reflect on what drives you toward this particular meal, snack, or nibble.

1. *Rate your* want *to eat.* On a scale of one to ten, how much do you want that food, that next bite? The number one represents a low level of desire and the number ten represents a high level of desire.

2. *Rate your* need *to eat.* On a scale of one to ten, how hungry are you? Remember, we're talking true physiological hunger, not appetite. The number one represents being uncomfortably stuffed, the midpoint of five represents being neither hungry nor full, and the number ten means you're experiencing intense physiological hunger. If you're not sure if you want to eat or need to eat, ask yourself the following three questions (ATE):

    A: Do I feel the *absence* of food in my stomach? (Is it growling?)

    T: Does the *time* suggest that it's likely I might be hungry? (For example, did you eat fifteen minutes or four hours ago?)

    E: Do I need this food for *energy*?

If you answered yes to all three questions, you're most likely experiencing physical hunger. Use this exercise as often as you need to until you identify the difference between hunger and appetite. Don't feel silly—it can take a while to distinguish between the two, especially if you're not used to doing it!

3. *Compare the two ratings.* Often this process shifts my clients into that *aha* place. They can step back and observe the difference between an emotional urge to eat and a basic need to refuel.

   If the want rating is higher than the need rating, pause. You may be acting on emotion rather than intellect. Give yourself at least ten seconds to think through your decision. (Count silently to ten if necessary.)

   As an example, let's say your want rating for a peanut butter cookie is high but your need rating is low. You may notice a very strong what-the-hell response. It's fine to eat a treat now and then, but if you acted on every high want rating, you'd be in trouble. This is an opportunity to reflect on the benefits of becoming more discerning about what you want. You may want a cookie or a brownie. But which do you want more? Unless you're ready to eat both, press PAUSE and think it through.

   If the need rating is higher than the want rating, eat. However, think before you reach. When you're really hungry, you'll eat whatever is convenient. In the long run, however, if food isn't very satisfying, you tend to continue to eat, searching for some pleasure—and that pleasure can quickly lead to regret.

   If the want and need ratings are essentially the same, eat! It's appropriate to eat when you're hungry. And it's a pleasure to eat when you're hungry *and* you like what you're eating, because you'll feel both physically and emotionally satisfied. But proceed with caution. When you're eating what you like *and* you're physically hungry, listen to your hunger and fullness cues.

Tool 7: The Mindful Bite

For the past few years, in my workshops on mindful eating, I've been teaching people to eat chocolate in a mindful way. (It may be more accurate to say that I teach the art of *savoring*.) But the real power of this mindful-eating exercise is in its use of chocolate rather than the traditional raisins or orange slices. Why? Because as any chocoholic knows, chocolate is a powerful trigger for emotion. Using chocolate illustrates perfectly the complexity of emotions we experience when we take a single bite.

In the following exercise, you'll tap into your emotional intelligence by paying attention to not just the sensations you experience, but also the feelings, thoughts, and memories that pop up. Being aware of the feelings and thoughts that swirl below the surface of your consciousness can give you insight as to why and how you crave chocolate.

The love of chocolate goes far beyond its taste. Yes, you love it, but what feelings come up as you eat it? In my previous books, I teach the *mindful bite*—the process of tuning in to your five senses as you eat a single bite of food. This tool—created specifically for people who like chocolate—takes the mindful bite a step further. As you savor a single bite of chocolate, this exercise invites you to notice how your feelings change from moment to moment, from the start of the bite to the end.

This is a powerful exercise—so powerful, in fact, that people who've taken my workshops more than once come up to me and tell me they think of me every time they unwrap a chocolate or see chocolate cake or ice cream. Although I've written this tool with chocolate in mind, you can practice it with any triggering food—chips maybe?—any food at all. But keep it to one bite. (If chocolate is a trigger food for you, you might ask a friend to sit with you while you do this exercise to ensure that you don't overeat it.)

You'll need a one-ounce piece of your favorite chocolate (still wrapped, if possible) and a ceramic plate of any size. Sit at the kitchen table at a quiet time when you're alone (perhaps at night, after everyone's in bed). If your favorite chocolate food is something other than bar chocolate, portion out one bite.

1. Place the wrapped chocolate (or the one bite) on the plate and take a seat.

2. Close your eyes and recall your most vivid memory of chocolate. Is it the dense, luscious chocolate layer cake your grandmother made on your birthday each year? The time you ate too much mousse and got miserably sick or felt extreme guilt and remorse? These are merely examples; dig deep and find that memory.

3. Tune in to your senses.

4. Now, if you're eating a piece of chocolate, unwrap it slowly. Listen to the crinkle of the paper. Close your eyes and hold the chocolate under your nose to inhale its fragrance. Rub your thumb across its smooth, unblemished surface. Inspect the chocolate, noticing its details. Is it light or dark? Can you detect the presence of crispies or caramel? Is the chocolate embossed with a pattern or dusted with nuts or sea salt? Then, and only then, place that one bite into your mouth and *taste it*. Chew it slowly, or let it melt in your mouth.

    If you're eating one bite of your favorite chocolate treat, follow the same process. Notice its color, texture, the direction in which the icing swirls, and other sensory details. Let no detail escape your notice. Then, and only then, place that one bite into your mouth and *taste it*. Chew it slowly, or let it melt in your mouth.

5. Answer the following questions, based on your experience from the beginning of the bite until the end.

    a. *Transience.* Did your desire for the chocolate change? Did it start strong and then fade by the time you finished the bite? Or did your desire intensify, so that by the end of the bite you wanted more?

    b. *Memories.* Describe any memories that came to mind—making fudge with your grandmother, a flourless chocolate torte from your favorite restaurant, sweets after school, etc. How did this memory shape your expectations of what you would taste and feel? Did it exceed or fall short of your expectations and hopes?

c. *Multiple Feelings.* Name the various feelings you experienced
    during the bite. Guilt? Pleasure? Desire? Did any one feeling
    overshadow the rest?

d. *Intensity.* How intense were the feelings you listed above? Were
    some strong and others subtle? Did you experience cravings?

e. *Judgment.* Did you find yourself judging what you felt? If so, did
    you deem those feelings okay or appropriate, or unacceptable
    or bad?

Many of my clients who've tried this tool are surprised by the complexity of the emotions they experience. However, feelings about other foods you love, especially those attached to vivid memories, can be just as complex—all the more reason to remember this experience the next time you eat chocolate or any other food that has an emotional pull. At that time, eat slowly and trail closely behind your feelings. See where they lead you before you take the next bite.

Tool 8: Open Mind, Closed Mind

"There exist limitless opportunities in every industry," said the American engineer Charles F. Kettering, inventor of the electric starter. "Where there is an open mind, there will always be a frontier."

Perhaps changing the way you eat is *your* new frontier to explore—and an essential tool for any type of exploration is open-mindedness. To be open-minded is to hope, to *believe* that we can change—if not the world, our own lives.

To achieve success in your life and relationships, it's essential to cultivate the EI quality of open-mindedness—to be intellectually curious, willing to seek new experiences and explore new ideas. These qualities are important for any entrepreneur, but no less important when you seek a new approach to managing your eating or your weight. With an open mind, you won't just think outside the box; you may not even *see* the box. That's how powerful the tool of open-mindedness is.

Openness is correlated with emotional intelligence. The more open you are to perceiving and acknowledging *all* your feelings—the good, the bad, and the ugly—the more effectively you'll manage them. For me, open-mindedness is when a client squares his or her shoulders and says, "I'm going to be honest with you" or "I'm not going to sugarcoat this." I know that person has taken the first step toward exploring positive alternatives.

By contrast, closed-minded people revert to their old ways of thinking and behaving—ways that didn't work then and won't work in the future. To me, closed-mindedness is when a client struggling with chronic stress tells me, "I was freaking out and needed chocolate." That's the end of the story— *that person's* story. Had he or she been open to accepting the stress in the moment—having perceived the feeling, sought a new way to manage the stress—he or she could have written a new ending to an old story: about freaking out and *not* eating the last chocolate éclair in the office kitchen.

To raise your Eat.Q., it's critical that you begin to view your feelings— even, and especially, the painful ones—as useful information. I'm remembering a scene from some TV show from my childhood, when a Native American guide put his ear to the ground, listened intently to the faint and distant rumble, and said, "This way!" Think of all your feelings as your Native American guide. When you take the time to listen to them, they'll guide you to true north.

In this exercise, you'll practice being open-minded. We often say (unconsciously, of course), "I don't want to feel (fill in the blank: stressed, tired, bored, angry, sad, lonely)." This exercise asks that you keep an open mind about these negative feelings and let them be your guide. Try it, and I'd be willing to bet that you won't use food to push down any of your feelings or experiences.

EXERCISE

1. Pick a day when you will commit to being open-minded. Choose a day that you know won't be overly stressful, with few commitments or deadlines.

2. On this day, go about your normal business. However, from the moment you open your eyes to the time you turn in, observe and notice any signs of closed-mindedness. Red-flag thoughts include:

   - *I don't want to.*

   - *It's not fair.*

   - *I don't want to feel that.*

   - *I don't like this.*

   - *No way.*

3. Stare down closed-minded thoughts. Explore them. Sift them through your mind. When your mind says *no,* respond with a statement that suggests that you will approach rather than shy away from them. Some sample responses to *no:*

   - *Yes!*

   - *I'll try.*

   - *I welcome it in.*

   - *I'll take a closer look.*

   - *This feeling is my guide, not my enemy.*

4. Follow up with three options. If chocolate is your go-to food for dealing with stress, think of three new options. You don't have to do them. Just open your mind to other options. You could go for a walk, return e-mails, or opt for a stress-relieving snack. If you can try one or all of these new options, great. If not, it's enough for now to train your mind to open rather than snap shut.

10

A

Accepting Your Emotions, Understanding Their Meaning

> Thinking is easy, acting is difficult, and to put one's thoughts
> into action is the most difficult thing in the world.
>
> —Johann Wolfgang von Goethe

The E tools strengthen your ability to perceive and welcome in *all* your feelings—the good, the bad, and the ugly—as you experience them. However, it does no good to welcome them in after you've polished off the ice cream. That welcoming must occur in the moment of decision, as you're wavering between what you *want* (or you believe will soothe painful or negative feelings) and what you *know*.

That's where the A tools come in. Their job is to help you begin to think about your feelings so you can understand and use them. Taken together, the A tools are a bridge that leads you from where you are (perceiving your feelings) to where you want to go (changing your behavior).

The bridge is thinking about your feelings. You may be wondering why this is necessary. Isn't knowing how you feel enough? While that's a good start, consider this: to manage your emotions and turn to positive alternatives, it's essential to understand how specific feelings affect *you*.

You're an original. Your history, temperament, gifts, and challenges are unique to you. The A tools help you discover more about who you are, so you can use this awareness to understand why your feelings affect you as they do. How do you cope with anger, stress, loneliness, fear? What specific situations, events, or people trigger these feelings, and along with them, the urge or desire to eat? How do you typically react to these feelings? What strengths do you possess that might help you change self-defeating thoughts and behaviors? By getting you to think about these and other questions, the A tools increase self-knowledge and self-awareness.

As you've learned, emotions are fleeting; they come, they go, one can slide quickly into another. The A tools also develop your capacity to shift your thinking as your feelings shift, so you can respond appropriately to any feeling rather than react to it.

Tool 9: Play to Your Strengths

Psychologist Howard Gardner, one of the first to view intelligence beyond the limits of IQ, once observed, "We all spend far too much time trying to remedy our weaknesses rather than building on our strengths." Absolutely, and I'd add that when it comes to our eating, we tend to dwell on what we do wrong rather than what we get right.

Part of building EI is learning to tune in to your strengths, whatever they are, in any situation. Knowing and acknowledging your strengths isn't pride; it's self-awareness. When I meet with clients, I immediately start looking for their strengths—and I always find some. Then I point them out, help the clients acknowledge them, and offer suggestions on how they might use them to improve their eating. If they're great researchers, I put them to work finding new recipes. If they're motivated by competition, I suggest forming a healthy-eating challenge with their coworkers. I recall one client who was an expert calligrapher. To reinforce a more positive way to think about food, I had her write empowering statements on thick, beautiful paper in her elegant script. I remember she chose a quote by Alexander Graham Bell: "When one door closes, another opens; but we often look so long and so regretfully upon the closed door that we do not see the one which has opened for us." This particular quotation helped her look for opportunities to eat better rather than mourn the loss of her old way of eating.

Emotionally intelligent people also acknowledge their weaknesses (although I don't like that word; I prefer *challenges*). Knowing and acknowledging that you tend to be impatient, procrastinate, or avoid confrontations will help you manage the emotions that arise when you're in situations that make you impatient, or you receive a work project with a deadline, or you must cope with an overbearing family member or coworker. And you know what that means: managing emotions is a sign of strength. So, by acknowledging your weaknesses, you're actually adding to your strengths!

In the context of eating, playing to your strengths while acknowledging your challenges helps you make insight-driven decisions. It's a Triple-P plan in action. Let's say you acknowledge that your Achilles' heel is eating at night. Once you say it aloud (perceive), you know (predict) that you typically make eating missteps between seven P.M. and bedtime. Knowing that, you can plan (prepare) most of your interventions for that time period. If chocolate leaves you cold but you swoon for fast food, you can put a Triple-P plan in place. To paraphrase that old adage, *self*-knowledge is power.

You don't necessarily have to "fix" the weakness; all you need to do is know how to minimize the damage or find ways to join your challenges with your strengths. For example, if you're a detail-oriented person and love lists, make a list of steps to tackle how you're going to avoid your junk-food cravings. It's also possible to turn your challenges into strengths. For example, if you're a night eater, why not make dinner your main meal of the day and resolve to make it the most nutritious?

When you play to your eating strengths, rather than get derailed by your challenges, food ceases to become the enemy. No matter how discouraged you feel about your eating or your weight, you do have strengths. You may have lost sight of them, however. The following exercise—a self-assessment of your strengths around food—helps you find them again.

EXERCISE

DAY 1

Your job is to let go of the negatives and setbacks and tune in to your strengths. These are the situations in which you shine, and these make you feel good about yourself. One might be eating a healthy breakfast or passing up a second treat. Whatever you do well in eating situations, jot it in your Eat.Q. notebook. You may also want to write on these prompts:

- I ate my healthiest meal at . . . (breakfast, lunch, dinner)
- The healthy foods I naturally love are . . .
- The snack that I love most (and don't binge on) is . . .
- I feel most proud when I eat . . .
- I find it easiest to eat well when I am . . .
- The biggest accomplishment in my life is . . .
- The skill that helped me with that accomplishment was . . .
- I can apply this skill to eating by . . .

DAY 2

Create one small goal that takes your strengths to the next level. If you found that breakfast was your healthiest meal of the day, add a piece of fruit or a handful of almonds to make it even healthier. If lunch was your favorite meal, your goal might be to shop for the ingredients you need to make your lunches healthy every day. If you feel most proud when you walk by the vending machine at work, make sure you'll be able to walk on by every day, by having your favorite pre-portioned snacks at work.

DAY 3

Now that your strengths are on your radar screen, consider joining with an ally who has opposite skills and strengths. Let's say you have difficulty getting and staying motivated. Team up with a coworker whom you know to be a good cheerleader. If you're more a big-picture person, join with a detail-oriented friend who can help you create a workout schedule and meal plan to document your progress.

Tool 10: Mental Makeover: Reframe That Feeling

One helpful way to cope with feelings is to look at them in a different way—to assign a fresh perspective. Psychologists call this technique *reframing*. Note that the goal of reframing isn't to change the emotion itself but how you relate to it. As the name suggests, reframing is like putting a new frame around an old picture. In reframing, you look for the meaning, opportunity, or benefit from the feeling, even when the feeling is negative. In this way, you raise the likelihood that you'll make insight-driven decisions.

Let's say you've had a horrible day at work. You're exhausted, angry, and overwhelmed by the mountain of paperwork that awaits you tomorrow morning. In other words, you're stressed—a very familiar feeling.

You can react as you have in the past, thinking, *I am done. I can't take these awful feelings. Eating is the only thing that will take them away—I can't help it.*

Or you can give that old picture—those familiar negative emotions—a new frame. You might say, *Here I am, stressed out again. It stinks. But I'm home now, in my comfort zone. I can kick off these heels, change into my comfy clothes, and read a few pages of my book to wind down from the day.*

In the past, psychologists frequently gave clients the advice to reframe their thoughts. We gave it with the understanding that it "just works," though we didn't fully understand how. But findings from a recent study suggest that reframing affects the brain, particularly the region that mediates food cravings.

My clients have learned that reframing their feelings can have a positive effect not just on their eating but also on the quality of their day-to-day lives. One of my clients recently lost her job as a teacher. She spent the first few days brooding over how her family was going to make it without her salary. In session, I had her reframe the situation. After some thought, she said, "I was always worried that I wasn't spending enough time with my own kids, and the guilt really got to me. Now I have the opportunity to really be there for them in a way I didn't before." Not only did she cope better, but her positive feelings also gave her more emotional energy to continue making smart eating decisions.

Use the following exercise whenever negative feelings are dragging you down or you can't let go of them. With each response, you'll put negative or worrisome feelings into perspective, which reduces their intensity and therefore your need to eat to escape them.

1. Sit in a comfortable chair. Close your eyes. Let your mind drift for a few moments.

2. When you feel ready, read the following list of questions. Which one jumps out at you? Reflect on it for a few moments.

   - Is there another feeling that could be worse than this one?

   - What else could this feeling mean beyond my first impression?

   - What might I learn from this situation?

   - What can I find that is humorous about this feeling?

   - What can I learn from this feeling to guide me?

   - What potential benefits or opportunities for growth might this feeling offer me?

   - How would one of my role models, heroes, or friends cope with this problem?

Tool 11: Try a Little Tenderness

Empathy—the ability to walk in someone else's shoes—is a critical emotional intelligence skill. The ability to tune in to and understand how someone else feels helps you communicate with that person effectively and connect on a deeper level. Ultimately, strong empathy skills lead to solid, lasting relationships and career success.

Empathy for yourself comes first—it's difficult to feel compassion for others, without judgment, unless you can give this gift to yourself. Unfortunately, when it comes to body weight, it's difficult to have empathy for your own experience. It's more common to feel guilt and be critical, to play what I call the *blame-shame game*. The automatic and habitual response is to judge yourself:

I'm fat.

I'm so stupid for eating that. I know better.

How could I have cheated on my diet? I'm so weak.

It's human nature to think that such harsh judgment would encourage us to change, but it doesn't. In an attempt to "fix" problems, our minds focus on what's missing rather than what's there.

The good news is that when clinicians use compassion and empathy while counseling people with weight loss, clients open up about their feelings, plus lose more weight, studies show. It makes sense. When someone offers you empathy instead of judgment, it helps you access your emotions, increasing your willingness to take a risk and talk about what you're *really* feeling. Clients tell me that when they feel judged by a family member or a doctor, they clam up, sometimes even lie about their weight-loss process because they're afraid their genuine feelings will be used as ammunition against them in the future.

Judgments move you away from your internal experience. In other words, you avoid feelings because you fear that your mind will scold you or you'll get caught up in negative feelings, such as shame, regret, and angst. And then you eat to stuff them down. When you're able to be open and honest, you can explore the ways in which you can lose weight—what works and what doesn't.

In the following exercise, you'll begin by accessing empathy for yourself, then progress to displaying it to someone else. You'll need your Eat.Q. notebook for this one.

EXERCISE

To begin this exercise, sit in a quiet, comfortable spot at a quiet time. Do some deep breathing, and let your mind wander. This would be a good opportunity to think about where you are at this moment in your journey toward healthy eating. Are you where you want to be? Are you satisfied or dissatisfied with your progress? Tune in to your self-talk. If you hear only negative chatter (*I have the willpower of a wet noodle. It's my own stupid fault I'm so heavy*), you're playing the blame-shame game.

In your Eat.Q. notebook, rewrite these statements with nonjudgmental words. Instead of blame and shame, think validate and support. For example, *It's okay. This is really hard. Keep trying, just for today.* These statements communicate an understanding that eating healthy and losing weight aren't easy and that not acing them right away doesn't mean you're stupid or incapable, just that you're human.

1. Practice at least once a day. When you start to notice and tune in to judgment, you may be surprised at how often you think something is critical.

2. After a few days, start to show empathy toward other people. For example, when you hear people chitchatting about food and dieting, focus on providing empathy, not a judgment ("You're on a diet. Do you really need that extra piece of pizza?") or advice ("*Here's* how you lose weight . . ."). Swap the words "good" and "bad" for nonjudgmental words, such as "healthy" or "skillful." If you can't be positive, be neutral ("It's okay."). To communicate empathy is as simple as saying, "It sounds like you feel . . ." and validating their feeling, whether it's frustration, anger, or sadness. You can also show empathy with your body: a nod of sympathy or a gentle touch on their arm or shoulder.

Attaining a healthy weight is important, but the process of getting there is rarely easy. Once you accept that, it gets easier to be gentle with yourself and show that same compassion and tolerance for others who are going through the same challenge.

Tool 12: Predict Your Emotional "Weather"

When the weatherperson says there's a chance of rain, I carry an umbrella. Of course, I've gotten drenched by the odd storm that blew in out of nowhere, but does that mean it's a waste of time to carry an umbrella when rain is predicted?

Of course not. Though the weatherperson sometimes gets it wrong, he or she also gets it right. The ability to predict how you'll feel in the future, as a weatherperson predicts the weather for the next week, is called *affective forecasting*. Wouldn't it be great if you could foresee how your choices will affect your future well-being? Well, you can. In fact, your expectations about emotional reactions to future events can help guide your decisions about relationships, career pursuits, and your eating.[1]

Affective forecasting is strongly linked to emotional intelligence, which makes sense. If you can "forecast" how you'll feel in the future, you can better prepare yourself for the "weather" of emotions, including those that drive your urge or desire to eat.

Let's say you have an exam or a big meeting two days from now. You can predict that you're likely to feel stressed and you prepare yourself—review your notes, get enough rest, eat well, psych yourself up with a running pep talk. Such preparation eases your stress and, by extension, reduces the likelihood that you'll overeat to soothe it.

You can also use affective forecasting to predict how you'll feel if you overeat. Yes, you have to train your mind to predict the consequences of an emotion-driven decision: *If I eat that, I'll feel bloated, miserable, and guilty, and I don't want to feel that way.* Evaluating how you are likely to feel after eating one too many slices of pizza takes practice, but that practice pays off in the moment of decision. Interestingly, in this case, your focus on avoiding the potentially negative immediate consequences—feeling bloated and miserable—outweighs the future benefits of weight loss.

When you do overeat, don't beat yourself up—guilt is a pretty useless emotion because it doesn't necessarily lead to behavior change. Rather, commit to memory how you felt physically (bloated, lethargic). Get really detailed. Remembering the sensory feelings that accompany overeating can help you use that experience later to make the connection between behavior and consequence. It will help you use the skill of affective forecasting: *When I ate X I felt X, and I don't want to feel X again.* In a sense, the memory and those sensory details are an emotional umbrella that will help protect you from emotional bad weather that leads to overeating.

In my experience, the clients who get good at emotional forecasting keep at it until the behavior–consequence connection is solid. At first, that connection is faulty: *I was about to eat a second slice of cake, predicted that I would feel guilty and overly stuffed, and I ate it anyway.* In time, it gets strong: *I was about to eat a second slice of cake, but I didn't because I didn't want to feel overly stuffed and guilty.* See the difference? The client got it in time.

You will too, and the following exercise will help you make that connection. I recommend practicing this several days in a row, whether or not you experience a desire or urge to eat. I also suggest writing these questions on an index card, laminating it, and reading the card when you're tempted to overeat. (Excuse yourself from the table if you must and find a private place to read and answer them.)

EXERCISE

Get out your Eat.Q. notebook. Write out the following questions, and then answer them. As you answer each question, get as specific as possible.

1. What am I likely to feel if I eat this? Be specific, particularly about the sensory feelings that accompany overeating (unbuttoning the top button of your jeans or loosening your belt, feeling gastrointestinal distress, waking up bloated the next day, and so forth).

2. Are these feelings likely to be positive or negative?

3. If I eat this, what is likely to be the difference between my initial feeling and the feeling I may experience several minutes later?

4. How long is the initial feeling likely to last? One minute? Five minutes? One day?

5. How intense will the initial feeling be on a scale from one to ten (one being not at all intense and ten being unbearably intense).

6. How long is the secondary feeling likely to last? One minute? Five minutes? One day?

7. How intense will the secondary feeling be on a scale from one to ten (one being not at all intense and ten being unbearably intense).

Tool 13: Take a "Time-In"

It's not always easy to integrate thought with feeling, especially when you're angry. In fact, anger is the cause of cases of DWE (deciding while emotional) a great deal of the time.

Think for a moment about how you express anger. Do you let it all out in a geyser of yelling and cursing? Push it down and let it fester? Fume silently as you think, resentfully, *I'll show you?* If any of those reactions sound like you, think about this: if anger isn't allowed outward expression, it turns inward, and *you're* the one who suffers.

Overeating is one expression of anger turned inward. Think about how your eating is affected when you're irritated or angry. How do these emotions affect your thinking? Do they raise or reduce your ability to think logically or motivate you to do better. One of my clients uses the word *pissivity*—a combination of *positivity* and *pissed off*—to explain that anger challenges her to do better. She embraces her anger, using it to fuel her workouts and make better choices. (*See, I can do it!* she says to herself.)

As counterintuitive as it sounds, a study published in the psychological journal *Emotion* suggests that it can be smart to get angry.[2] In this study of 136 people, mostly women, those who *wanted* to be angry during a confrontation were found to be higher in EI than those who wanted to be happy during a conflict. Those okay with being angry understood that being upset during a conflict is the "right" feeling. If you don't welcome in the anger, it's likely that you might let go of an important issue. Perhaps you might tell yourself it's not that big of a deal or to just forget about it. My experience tells me that you won't forget about it. In fact, it's highly likely that you'll DWE—raid the refrigerator, hit the vending machine, pull up to the drive-through. While it can be smart to get angry, it's rarely smart to act in the heat of it.

In many situations, emotions can help guide your next action. (I've heard it explained as "doing the next right thing.") Let's say that you've just hung up on your cable provider after an angry dispute about a bill and you're about to make dinner. You open the freezer and rummage around angrily. Will it be a stir-fry, as you'd planned, or—the hell with it—the frozen pizza you keep for your teenage boy, who's hungry at odd hours? If you welcome in that anger and acknowledge that it's driving you to DWE, you can take a different action that will help you discharge your anger in a more positive and much more effective way. Pizza may numb the anger, but it won't get rid of it the way making a phone call to a friend to vent might.

Whether it's anger or sadness, it's imperative to stick with your uncomfortable feelings, thinking about them and deciding on a productive solution. We often teach kids to do a "time out" when they're overwhelmed by their feelings of anger. In this exercise, you will be doing a "time in" to tune in to your anger. Instead of taking a break from your anger, this exercise invites you to take a few minutes to zero in on it. You'll need a simple kitchen timer for this one.

EXERCISE

1. The next time you're angry, set the timer for five minutes.

2. Do the Q-TIPP (focused breathing) exercise in chapter 2 to calm the physiological components of anger (reduce your heart rate, increase oxygen flow).

3. While you're angry (don't try to suppress it!), listen to what it's telling you. Specifically, in that five minutes, outline in your head what is *useful* about this emotion. What does it tell you about the next action to take? If you need to, remind yourself you're experiencing anger in this moment for a good reason. Your job is to find that reason rather than lose it in food.

4. When the timer dings, commit to taking one action step to manage your anger in a positive way. Journal about it, call someone to talk it out, meditate, go to the gym, steam-clean the carpet. By now, you've learned that you have options; your next step is to pick one.

Tool 14: Give Habits the Slip

We overeat for many reasons, but a biggie is plain old habit. Habit is a behavior that occurs automatically; we really don't even think about it. We have many habits, and some are healthy, such as eating breakfast every morning before leaving for work, which research indicates is one of the best ways to start the day and maintain your weight. Some habits are not so healthy, such as a regular late-night snack right before bed. When I begin working with a client, one of our first steps is to identify and differentiate between eating that is intentional (actively choosing to eat) and eating that the person has just slipped into without even knowing it (mindlessly munching). It can help people stop being so hard on themselves. In some ways, changing a habit is quite challenging, because you first have to catch yourself doing it—realizing that you slip into munching when you're bored, for example. But catching yourself interrupts how the habit plays out. It's like changing the direction of the flow of a stream. The good news is that habits are very malleable. You can change them, and doing so makes life a lot easier.

By definition, habits are predictable. Your significant other can likely choose what you'll pick on a menu, what you're likely to bring home from the supermarket, or what you'll choose for a midnight snack. Habits that lurk below your awareness won't budge. You have to bring them out into the light of day. Once you become conscious of your habits, it's hard not to notice them. People who are emotionally intelligent tap into their self-awareness and closely examine how their behavior can railroad them time and again into unhealthy decisions.

A key place to start is to focus less on breaking old negative habits and more on forming positive new ones. I see my clients struggle and fight with themselves to break old habits. But when they build up a new healthy habit, it often alters the unhealthy habit with little effort and less frustration. It's hard to drink four sugary beverages a day when you add a salad and a piece of fruit to both your lunch and dinner. You'll naturally gravitate to a beverage that complements your new, positive eating habits.

A study published in the *European Journal of Social Psychology* recruited ninety-six people to investigate how long it took them to form a new habit.[3] The researchers wanted to discover if eating a piece of fruit with lunch or going for a fifteen-minute run each day could become a behavior that people did with little or no effort. Each day participants recorded how automatic the behavior was. In other words, was it "hard not to do" and was it done "without thinking." Although outcomes ranged from 18 days up to 254 days, on average it took 66 days for these behaviors to turn over into a habit requiring little or no effort.

Thus, the good news is that you can build healthy habits. The challenge is doing the same behavior repeatedly for two solid months. The benefit of sticking with it is that the healthy behaviors you want will become part of your new routine. If you skip a day, the study said it was "okay. It didn't matter that much." Also, it's important to keep in mind that easier, simple behaviors (say, adding an apple) take less time to change than complex behaviors that take more effort (cooking a meal, for example).

EXERCISE

1. Do an observational study of your habits. Write them down in your Eat.Q. notebook as soon as you notice them. Some you may be very aware of, such as eating while watching TV or using a one-for-you-one-for-me strategy when making a snack for your child. Others may not be as obvious because they happen only in certain circumstances, such as buying sweets every time you get on an airplane. Just becoming more conscious of your habits can begin the process of shifting them.

2. Build new habits. In your Eat.Q. notebook, choose just one good habit to focus on. Here are some ideas:

   • Swap fizzy drinks for water.

   • Don't work, read, drive, or do anything else when you eat.

   • Bring a piece of fruit or a small fruit salad to work to snack on each day.

   • Serve meals from the stove rather than put the serving dishes on the table (it's harder to take seconds).

   • Sit down when you eat—for example, don't stand next to the open refrigerator and nibble from containers of food.

   Are you unsure which good habit to tackle first? A study in the *Archives of Internal Medicine* found that changing two simple habits—eating more fruits and vegetables and cutting back on TV time—can result in a big positive effect.[4]

3. Each day, rank the ease of the habit from one to ten (one being easy to integrate into your life and ten being impossible). Some good habits may take a week to master; others will take longer. That's okay. Just keep plugging away. When you've completely integrated that good habit into your life, begin another.

As you integrate new habits into your life, periodically evaluate whether your old habits have begun to shift in a positive direction. If one or more persist, they've become engrained behavior. One solution is to throw a monkey wrench into your routine. For example, when eight P.M. rolls around and your habit is to get a snack, lie on the sofa, and pick up the remote, mix it up. Sit on a chair or even the floor. In this new location, you might still eat the snack, but it will feel slightly different, which is what you want. The change makes you more conscious of your behavior—perhaps enough to think it through and stop it.

Another tactic to try is to remove the reinforcing nature of a habit. We develop habits because they feel good. Changing the expected or usual outcome of a habit can help you break it. The idea is to take the pleasure down a notch. Eat standing up. Have the pancakes without the butter. Get a brand of crisps that are just "okay" instead of your favorite crinkle-cut brand. It can actually be rather fun to think outside the box to find ways to short-circuit your own bad habits.

Tool 15: Squash Your Desire to Emotionally Eat—Write Away

I always smile when I see clients come in with a journal tucked under their arms. I know that they are making important connections between how they feel and what they eat.

Journaling is a key way to develop your emotional intelligence. Journaling is not simply recording the events of your day. It's about exploring your thoughts *and* feelings about those events. In this case, the focus is on the specific feelings that drive you to food.

In a way, the time spent writing in your journal is a mindful pause that allows you to express your feelings in any words you choose. Later, that raw emotion gives you the opportunity to think about how you use food and why (to calm yourself, numb out, or express particular emotions, such as anger).

If you're anything like my clients, you may feel resistance to the thought of journaling. Maybe you're concerned that you don't have time, or you fear that what you write won't be "good enough," or you won't be able to put what you feel into words. But can you keep an open mind? Are you willing to try it for a week? You don't have to write pages and pages to get remarkable insights into your eating. You just have to be honest. And because no one else will be reading your journal, it's safe to write the truth.

Science has shown that when people put experiences into words it can help mitigate the physical effects of stress. In a study of 122 students conducted at the University of Iowa, researchers examined the effect of writing about a traumatic event. The researchers had one group of students journal about the emotions related to the event, one group write about their emotions *and* their thoughts, and one group write factually about that day's news. Notice that the second group didn't just list their day-to-day experiences, which is a cognitive task. They focused on making sense of their experience—an emotional processing task. This difference is similar to the IQ–Eat.Q. divide—it's not what you know; it's what you know about *how you feel*.

Interestingly, while writing about emotions alone increased negative symptoms from the trauma, study participants who recorded both thoughts and feelings developed a sense that the trauma had produced some positive effects in their lives.[5]

At the end of the day, we are all simply trying to make sense of our experiences. And many of our interactions with food and feelings don't make sense at first glance. For example, one of my clients wrote, "Stuffed myself with cookies right out of the oven. I told myself to stop, and then said, 'What the hell.' Two hours later, I hate myself." However, her cookie binge didn't hit out of the blue. From her journal entries, she could see that it had actually begun two days before, when she'd started yet another diet. The decision to diet was prompted by seeing an ex-boyfriend with another girl, which had devastated her. She was jealous of the new girlfriend's slender figure. *Maybe he wanted me to be thin like her,* she thought. So, she went on a diet. However, swearing off sugar led to intense cravings, which led to the cookie binge. No sugar, a hurtful encounter with an ex . . . there was more than a simple desire for cookies going on. Her journal had taught her an important lesson: there's almost always a reason you overeat, but you have to trace it to the root cause.

Many people prefer the vintage paper-and-pencil journal, but feel free to tap out your thoughts on your desktop or laptop or at an online journaling site. Use whatever method feels right and best reveals your emotions.

There is no right way to keep a food journal, but most people list the following items each time they eat:

- *When.* The time you noticed the emotion or ate.

- *Where.* Your whereabouts when the eating occured, and whom you were with, if anyone.

- *Hunger Level.* Rated on a scale of one to ten (one being not at all hungry and ten being ravenous).

- *Food.* What you ate; be specific and honest, but this item isn't your main focus.

- *Emotion Before Eating.* How you felt before you ate, making your description as honest and detailed as possible.

- *Emotion After Eating.* How you felt after you ate, making your description as honest and detailed as possible.

As you write, focus on how you felt, not on what or how much you ate. You're delving into what's going on before, during, and after you eat and your emotions around eating. Notice the connections, if any, between how you felt before and after you ate, and the specific emotions that prompted you to eat.`

EXERCISE

- Devote a section of your Eat.Q. notebook to a seven-day journal.

- Journal each day, at the same time (many of my clients like to journal in the quiet part of the evening, a few hours before bedtime), using the guidelines above. Write as much or as little as you wish, but hit all the bullet points above.

- Don't edit your thoughts; write from the heart. You're not journaling to censor your feelings but to feel and process them.

Another option, if you would like more structure, is to use the template that follows. Identify the most significant event of your day—the event you feel compelled to write about. It may be about food (discussing dinner with your family over the holidays) or not (a frustrating day at the office). Then follow the EAT method model.

E: *Embrace* and tune in. Describe the event in detail and at least two feelings that accurately describe how you feel about the event.

A: *Accept* these feelings, whether negative or positive. Are you struggling against them in any way? How so? Are you pushing them away, avoiding them, clinging to them? Or are you simply accepting them as they are?

T: *Turn to* what can you do to make the situation better. Make a list of actions you can take (get out of the situation, exercise, call someone).

Tool 16: Dig In to a Therapeutic Dose of Produce

When stressed, most people turn to food that's packed with sugar, salt, and fat. There's no doubt that comfort foods do comfort—momentarily. Soon after the last bite, however, they can trigger an emotional eating "hangover" of regret and guilt, worsened by physical symptoms such as bloat and fatigue.

It doesn't have to be that way. A recent study suggests that fruits and vegetables—rather than ice cream, nachos, or macaroni and cheese—may actually promote the positive, mood-altering benefits that comfort foods only seem to provide in the short term.

Researchers in New Zealand had 281 college students complete a daily food diary online. For twenty-one days, the students logged in to their diaries each night and rated how they felt from a list of eighteen words—nine positive and nine negative. The nine negative words included *depressed, sad, anxious, angry,* and *short-tempered.* The nine positive-affect adjectives included *calm, content, relaxed, happy,* and *excited.*[6]

The students also answered five questions about what they had eaten that day, including the number of servings of fruit (excluding juices and dried fruit), vegetables (excluding juices), and foods like cookies, crisps, and cake.

After three weeks, researchers analyzed both the diaries and the word choices. The results showed a strong day-to-day relationship between positive mood and a higher intake of fruits and vegetables, but not other foods. Specifically, on days when the students ate more fruits and vegetables—seven or eight servings a day—they reported feeling calmer and happier, with more energy. (That might sound like a lot of produce, but one serving can fit in the palm of your hand.) Thus, the therapeutic dose to see an improvement in mood wasn't just an apple a day—it was seven or eight servings.

To understand which came first—the positive moods or the intake of fruits and veggies—the team ran additional analyses. They found that eating fruits and vegetables predicted improvements in positive mood the next day. It wasn't clear whether the improvement in mood was due to the chemical properties—vitamins and minerals—or if it was because we tend to feel better when we make healthy choices.

So while baby carrots, fresh berries, or a juicy tomato don't have the taste and texture of traditional comfort foods, they may actually give you what you're seeking: a brighter mood. The exercise that follows is an investment in your mood. You'll need a simple calendar for this one.

EXERCISE

1. Purchase three of your favorite fruits and vegetables (I'd pick blueberries, fresh sugar snap peas, and either cantaloupe or sweet red and yellow bell peppers). Wash, peel, chop, and place them in plastic bags or containers. Your goal is to eat seven or eight servings a day, as the students in the study did, for the next five days. That's a doable amount—a handful of berries at breakfast, a salad at lunch, a cup of steamed veggies at dinner, a piece of fruit as a bedtime snack.

2. Place the calendar where you'll see and use it—on the kitchen counter or on the refrigerator door. Each day, at the end of the day, jot down two things: the number of servings of fruits and vegetables you ate and your day's mood from one to ten (ten being your brightest mood). Jot down, too, whether you engaged in stress eating, as well as how many times. (Focus on the positive, too. You're not *stopping* stress eating; you're *starting* healthy eating!)

3. Commit to the exercise for the five days. If you don't experience a positive effect on your mood or stress eating in the first day or two, hang in there. You just might see the benefits the next day.

4. At the end of five days, review your data. On the days you ate more fruits and veggies, did your mood seem to improve? If not, did it seem to be better the day after you ate more produce? Did you seem to manage your eating or your stress better?

11

T

Turning to New, Positive Alternatives to Eating

Freedom is the right to choose: the right to create
for oneself the alternatives of choice.

—Archibald MacLeish

The E and A tools develop your capacity to perceive and accept your feelings, respectively. To use that newfound understanding of your emotions, to manage them in the moment, you need the T tools. These tools invite you to think about the emotion you're experiencing *as you feel it,* so you can make a conscious choice about how you will respond. That awareness, and acceptance, is the raw material of insight-driven decisions. When you feel that you *must* eat, using one of the following tools can help you "surf" the feeling or dampen its intensity, so at the moment of decision you can press PAUSE and make an insight-driven choice.

That pause is critical, especially if you struggle with feelings that eat you up inside, such as shame, guilt, or anger. Maybe you ignore these feelings or bottle them up until they explode. Either way, not giving them the consideration they deserve can trigger cravings, overeating, or binges. The T tools lead you to a mindful pause, a conscious choice, and the ability to do something different when eating feels like the only possible option: you *respond* rather than react.

Because eating is so often an ingrained response to feeling, it takes time to learn new responses. Don't let setbacks discourage you. With practice, the new, empowering response (thinking about your feelings in the moment and using that information constructively) will become as ingrained as the old, destructive response (giving up and giving in).

The T tools give you the freedom to make a conscious decision to eat, or not. If your eating feels out of control, they offer you something you may have never known you had: a choice.

Tool 17: Taming Your Impulses

I want a cake!

More french fries!

Just another bite!

Do these demands sound familiar? All represent the inner voice that, when faced with pleasurable food, eggs you on. This voice doesn't always insist on extra pizza or M&M's before bed; it demands the satisfaction of other immediate desires (*I want to stay home from work, drive fast, gamble*). My clients often blame this voice for many of their impulsive eating decisions, such as giving in to cravings and overeating pleasurable foods. This inner voice is powerful and it can often feel as if it's in the driver's seat and you're just along for the ride. Maybe you've felt hopeless that this could ever change. Let's take a step back and understand why it's so hard.

Impulses begin in the prefrontal cortex, the part of your brain that makes decisions. There are two areas involved in impulsive behavior. The dorsolateral prefrontal cortex is in charge of making a plan, and choosing and suppressing urges. The orbitofrontal cortex is involved in managing emotions. Both areas quickly weigh the *now* versus *later* equation: Do you want a small payoff (a slice of cake) now or a bigger reward (weight loss) later? Often we impulsively opt for the immediate payoff and regret it later.

It doesn't help that preliminary research suggests that, compared to average-weight people, those who are overweight may be less able to shut off regions of the brain that drive food cravings. Their brains are more sensitive to food rewards. In a small study of nine normal-weight and five overweight people, researchers at Yale University and the University of Southern California scanned areas of the brain that activate when a person views pictures of tempting foods (burgers and fries, chocolate, ice cream), low-calorie foods (salads, broccoli, tofu), and common non-food items (a book, a bicycle, a door).

The volunteers' brains were scanned two hours after a meal, and the researchers purposely tweaked the subjects' blood sugar levels, scanning when their subjects had both normal and low blood sugar.

When blood sugar levels were low, brain "reward regions" lit up—signaling the desire to eat—and the prefrontal cortex was less able to put the brakes on these "Eat!" signals. This was especially true in the overweight volunteers when they viewed the pictures of tempting high-calorie foods. When blood sugar levels were normal, however, the scans of the normal-weight volunteers showed more activity in the prefrontal cortex, which reduced activity in their brains' reward regions.[1]

What's the bottom line? Fighting an impulse to eat is hard enough, so it's important to regulate your blood sugar. Restricting food causes cravings and the perceived reward factor is going to be big—much bigger than if your blood sugar levels were normal.

Happily, other research suggests that teaching your brain to recognize and handle your impulses may help quash impulsive eating. Researchers call this *inhibitory training*—the practice of engaging the brain regions responsible for stopping action. The more you work them, the stronger they get. For example, in a study conducted by Dutch researchers, chocolate lovers were divided into three groups and shown pictures of chocolate. The first group was given an inhibitory training task to perform as they viewed the pictures. (The task? Not to press a computer key.) The second group was asked to respond (to press the key) as they viewed the pictures. A control group responded to the pictures only during half the trials. After viewing the pictures, the volunteers were invited to eat chocolate. Those who performed the inhibitory task ate less chocolate than the other two groups, suggesting that practicing and engaging in inhibitory tasks helps.

What this finding suggests is that you have more power over your impulses than you think. With practice, the following exercise can help short-circuit your impulse to eat.

EXERCISE

This exercise is simple—but it isn't easy, especially in the beginning! It's well worth the practice, however. This exercise can give you enough time to respond rather than react to your immediate want and realize you've arrived at the moment of decision.

STEP 1

1. Listen for your *I want* voice.

2. Press PAUSE (page 47).

STEP 2

You can do your own inhibitory training. We use it all the time with kids because it works. They are taught to raise their hands before talking in school. Kids must line up before going out at breaktime instead of running wildly through the hall. In other words, these actions are evidence that we can teach ourselves to keep our impulses in check.

Throughout the day, create moments in which you intentionally hold back. An easy way to do this is to play Simon Says. This simple game perfectly mimics what it feels like to hold back—to restrain your impulses. The point is to teach yourself to say "stop," and then do it. We often don't think we have the power to stop eating once we start. This exercise shows you that you do. Practice the following tasks once or twice a day:

1. As you walk, say "Stop" aloud. Stop in your tracks for a moment, and then resume walking.

2. Drink a glass of water and, at random, pause for a moment. Then resume your drink.

3. Consciously adjust the length of time between the first moment you notice wanting something and giving it to yourself—whatever it may be—a snack, a break at work, checking your e-mail. Start with a minute. Then increase the length of time between noticing you want a snack and giving it to yourself.

Tool 18: Empowering Words

Say the following statements aloud:

> I can't have ice cream.

> I choose not to eat ice cream right now.

Quite a difference in meaning, isn't there? The first statement implies that you've run up against an external barrier—like a diet—that prevents you from partaking. The second implies that you've made a personal, internal choice not to partake.

The word *can't* is small but mighty; it wields great power. So do words like *should, ought to,* and *must.* They're black-and-white words that imply all-or-nothing thinking. Pit them against a craving or the urge to eat, and more often than not the craving or urge wins. I observe this with my clients frequently. Those who use such words struggle more with cravings and overeating than those who've excised these words from their vocabularies (typically, after we've begun EAT method work).

The words you choose matter, particularly those you use when you talk to yourself. The chatter and commentary inside your head can mean the difference between making a diet-derailing, emotion-driven decision, or an insight-driven decision that keeps your healthy diet on track.

Telling yourself you "should" choose healthy options, issuing yourself demands to "eat right!" or saying that you "can't" have a treat doesn't work. In fact, such tough talk can backfire. In a series of experiments published in the *Journal of Consumer Research,*[2] researchers broke 209 people into two groups. They had one group choose either a chocolate bar or an apple before they read a "controlling message" that they "should," "ought," "must," and/ or "need to" exercise. The other group was able to choose their snack after they read the message.

Those who exhibited self-control and chose the apple got testy when they read the message. Having mustered the self-restraint to choose the healthier snack, they didn't appreciate being told what they "ought" to do. The message irritated those who chose the chocolate too, just not as much as those who opted for the apple. That's probably because they chose the snack they wanted, and the one that didn't require them to exert self-control. Respond to temptation with the thought *I don't* instead of *I can't*. You may be more likely to resist it, according to another study published in the *Journal of Consumer Research*. In one of four experiments designed to test the power of *I don't* versus *I can't* thoughts, researchers randomly assigned 120 volunteers to one of two groups and gave each group a different strategy to resist temptation. The first group was instructed to think *I can't;* the second, *I don't*. To "rehearse" their strategies, the volunteers were given the example of being tempted by an unhealthy snack and thinking either *I can't eat X* or *I don't eat X*. Then they began a different and unrelated activity.

When the experiment was over, the researchers gave their volunteers a parting gift: either a granola bar or a chocolate bar. The *I don't* group chose the granola bar more often than the *I can't* group.

The findings suggest an age-old truth: we don't like anyone telling us what to do, including ourselves. When you're already exercising self-restraint (refusing a piece of homemade pie, choosing a salad over fries), it's more empowering to tell yourself you *don't* eat pie or fries and link that choice to an internal reason, rather than tell yourself you *can't* eat pie or fries because an external barrier stands in your way. People who use their emotional intelligence are typically quite thoughtful with their choice of words. For example:

> I can't eat ice cream because my class reunion is in two weeks (external cause).

> I don't eat ice cream because I don't want to sabotage my goals (internal cause).

When you're already trying to make positive changes, it's essential to find just the right words to empower and encourage you rather than deflate and discourage you.

1. *Catch negative chatter.* Tune in to your self-talk, especially when it's time for a meal or snack. Look especially for the words *must, can't,* and *should.* For example:

    I must not eat a second slice of pizza.

    I shouldn't eat those chips.

2. *Flip into an empowering statement.* Flip that negative self-talk into an empowered refusal. For example:

    I choose not to eat another slice of pizza.

    I don't eat chips because I choose not to.

Hear the difference? You're identifying your decision not to indulge as a choice from within rather than a demand forced on you by a diet or orders.

Tool 19: Eat.Q. "Yoga"

Your child wakes up with the flu the day the family is flying to Disney World. A storm leaves you stranded in the airport en route to a critical meeting. How do you cope with change? When your routine is messed with, when your plans go awry, do you sink or swim? More to the point, do you adapt or eat?

Flexibility is the ability to adapt and respond to change. How easily you can move from plan A to plan B is a hallmark of emotional intelligence, specifically the ability to manage the emotions that change can leave in its wake: frustration, anger, surprise.

I have clients who struggle with this crucial ability to adapt. Even small changes in their routines can wreak havoc on their eating. They may experience a small "slip" and be unable to get back on plan, or they have strict eat-this-don't-eat-that rules. One client actually passed up a piece of the birthday cake her daughter had made for her. Sadly, for psychologically inflexible people, that kind of behavior is par for the course. They're either following a punishing diet (until some situation or event triggers a binge) or overeating.

It's too bad, because flexibility is one of the emotional skills that factors into weight-loss success, research says. Researchers at the University of Würzburg in Germany compared people with a rigid approach to weight loss, who had strict dietary rules, to those with a flexible style, who tended to control portions and adjust how much they ate from day to day. All 616 participants experienced cravings. However, cravings were linked with difficulty in losing weight only for those with the strict eating approach.

It's possible that rigid dieters are more prone to a loss of control, the study said. However, while both groups sometimes gave in to cravings, flexible eaters may be more inclined to compensate by adjusting how much they eat afterward.[3]

Here are some other examples of circumstances that call for flexibility in eating:

- You packed a healthy lunch but a colleague you'd like to know better asks you to lunch.

- You're called out of town and you don't have access to the healthy foods you typically eat.

- A restaurant doesn't offer your regular option (say, you always order grilled fish and roasted potatoes) or one that's as healthy as you'd like.

Consider the examples above. Faced with each experience, would you adapt (go to lunch with the colleague and order a healthy entrée, wing it while you're out of town, go for the least calorie-laden entrée at the restaurant), or would the emotions triggered by the change cause you to eat more than you'd like or blow it completely? If the latter, just admitting that you tend to resist change is a good first step. Only then can you let go of plan A, accept plan B, and manage your emotions long enough to make a smart eating decision.

Not a go-with-the-flow type? That's okay. The following two-step exercise will help you stretch your ability to tolerate disruptions in your schedule. Think of it as Eat.Q. "yoga." It may be a bit uncomfortable, as limbering up your muscles can be, but before long you'll increase your mental flexibility enough to embrace plan B, stay strong, and make smarter decisions.

EXERCISE

STEP 1

For the next week, look for opportunities to change your daily routine—let's call it your plan A. The changes can be simple or complex, or a mix of both—your choice. To get you thinking, you might start your week of change by sitting in a different chair at your dining table (simple), progress to taking a walk around the block after dinner instead of heading to the TV (slightly harder), and end the week by mapping out a new route to work (complex). These are just examples; tailor your changes to your comfort level, and take all the time you need.

As you make these changes, be aware of the resistance you encounter within yourself—the uneasiness, fear, perhaps even panic. Struggling against such feelings uses up all your emotional energy. When you accept the feelings, you can devote your full attention to managing them.

So, embrace these feelings. Acknowledge that you prefer your plan A. Then say to yourself, *I welcome plan B*. This simple statement can help you manage that initial resistance to change.

STEP 2

When you feel ready, write out a detailed plan about what you will eat that day. Then, make one spontaneous change. It doesn't have to be dramatic. If you always eat a banana for a snack, choose an apple. If you usually order iced tea with lunch, opt for a glass of water with lemon. If you typically order fries, have a salad.

This tool helps you learn to adapt and be flexible to a change in plans without letting the emotions that accompany the change (fear, disappointment, confusion) overwhelm you. It also allows you to take change for a test drive. Although you're making a change, you're making it on your terms, so you still feel in control.

Repeat this exercise at least once a week, changing up things as your confidence grows. I'm betting that the next time you forget your carefully packed lunch at home, you won't panic and make an unhealthy choice.

Tool 20: The Craving Block

If you're like most people, you've been blindsided by cravings. There you are, lying on the sofa, innocently watching TV, when an intense craving strikes out of the blue. Imagining the object of your desire, in all its luscious, gooey, creamy, salty, or crunchy detail, is sucking up all your attention and energy.

Then you get a phone call—a welcome distraction from the craving. Much later, you notice that the desperate, gotta-have-it urgency is gone. That's the *elaborated intrusion theory of desire* in action.

In psychology, this theory suggests that our thoughts about food can ramp up our cravings. Especially when those thoughts lead to more elaborate thoughts—accompanied by vivid sensory images—about how to get what we desire. As it turns out, when it comes to cravings, mental pictures are key.

The theory works like this: Out of the blue, you think of a cinnamon roll. You briefly consider this unexpected thought and decide you want one. Of course, you don't have one, and your thoughts of the roll—and your mental pictures of it—become increasingly elaborate. Those mental pictures throw your senses into overload—the roll's buttery, sweet flavor; how easily the soft dough yields to your teeth; the soft, sweet heart of the roll, savored last.

All these vivid sensory images, each more elaborate than the last, help morph that unexpected thought into a full-blown craving.

A study conducted in the United Kingdom began with the hypothesis that food imagery plays a key role in cravings.[4] In two separate experiments, the researchers set out to test the hypothesis. In the first ten-minute experiment, they instructed volunteers to either "let their minds wander" or make cubes and pyramids out of modeling clay, alternating the shapes as quickly as possible. The clay squashers experienced fewer chocolate cravings than the daydreamers.

In the second experiment, researchers compared the effects on craving of a simple verbal task (counting by ones) versus working with clay. Again, clay won the day—the modelers reported that their cravings weakened, and they thought less often about chocolate.

How can pushing clay around short-circuit cravings? It's the elaborated intrusion theory in action: when you interrupt the mind's elaborating on the sensory aspects of a craved food—imagining the sweet taste, the creamy texture—the craving diminishes.

You can use the exercise explained in this study exactly as it's described. In this case, you'll need two lumps of modeling clay—one to use at work and one for home. You'll use the clay to direct your thoughts away from vivid sensory images of the food you're craving.

EXERCISE

- When a craving hits, work with your clay for ten minutes, as the subjects in the study did. You can make the shapes they made or use your imagination. By engaging your working memory on a specific task, you can reduce your mental imagery of the craved food and thus cool the craving.

- If you're caught without your clay, count backwards by three. According to the study, this simple task may engage your working memory enough to reduce cravings.

- If you don't want to work with clay, choose a pleasant but vivid non-food visual image (a green meadow, waves breaking on a beach).

Tool 21: Believe It, Achieve It

Have you ever said to yourself, "Why bother eating healthier? There is no way I am going to be able to change. I've tried. It didn't work then and it won't work now." My clients often come in with what I call "I surrender" thoughts. These "I surrender" thoughts come in lots of different forms, such as, "Oh well, I'm just destined to be this way." Or the what-the-hell thoughts begin to emerge—"I might as well have the ice cream. I always blow my diet." I understand. These thoughts spring out of frustration and fatigue.

Regardless, "I surrender" thoughts are very sneaky. They put a dramatic halt on your actions and are akin to putting on the breaks. When I hear these "I surrender" thoughts, I turn directly to the incremental beliefs theory to help me get my client back on track. In fact, believing that you have the power to make a change in yourself and situation is so critical that if I get wind that the "I surrender" thoughts are present, I stop right there and tackle them before we take even one more step forward.

The incremental beliefs theory is a complex term for a simple attitude. The theory posits that learning and effort can ultimately be fruitful—they lead to change. You have the capacity to learn and grow. According to this way of thinking, you can embrace change, persist when you have a setback, and see your efforts as a path to mastery, not a final destination.

Studies have even shown that reminding people of their capacity to change can act as a buffer or "vaccinate" them against giving up when they do slip up.[5] In other words, if you are eating well and then suddenly you mindlessly overeat, reminding yourself of the capacity for change can help prevent you from saying, "Oh, what the hell, I messed up anyway—might as well go all the way."

Incremental beliefs are tied in with emotional intelligence because EI helps people be open and flexible. I teach my clients how to use elements of this theory all the time. Clients initially come in with a subconsciously or consciously ingrained belief that nothing can change. If they believe that, nothing can or will change, including their ability to pick and choose healthy foods and to eat in a mindful way. But the opposite is true as well. The bottom line is that your mind-set does matter.

We all need concrete reminders that our world is fluid, flexible, and ever-changing. It isn't static even if it feels that way. Your surroundings are always changing and so are you. Remind yourself of this often. Embrace it. Use this knowledge as a tool to help you get back on track when your thoughts want to shut down your effort.

EXERCISE

- Listen closely for the *what the hell* in your head. When you hear it, don't fight it. Instead, say to yourself, either silently or aloud, "My eating isn't set in stone. I can change it. Hard work and effort make a difference."

- Think of someone you know who has successfully changed his or her eating habits. If that person did it, so can you.

- Set up a daily e-mail, delivered to yourself, with the subject heading "Healthy eating is obtainable." In the body of the e-mail, write something like "It's not the hand you're dealt that matters. It's how you play the hand." Write yourself a different e-mail every day, if you'd like, all with the same general message: food choices are changeable, and you can change yours. The daily e-mail will anchor this information in your mind and act as a daily "booster shot" against what-the-hell thinking.

Tool 22: Cash Only, Please

In line to order coffee, your eye falls on the glass case of pastries. When your turn comes, you order the coffee and hesitate. Those croissants look so plump, so soft, so sweet. Impulsively, you add a croissant to your order and hand over your debit card.

Sound familiar? Sometimes we eat unhealthy foods because our nutritional knowledge isn't up to date. All too often, however, it's because we want what we want. We see, we smell, and we whip out our debit or credit card.

Such impulsivity, fueled by emotion-driven decisions, seems to be one of the biggest influences on unhealthy food consumption. In fact, consumer research suggests that we use credit or debit cards more often than cash to buy "vice products," such as sugary coffee drinks, doughnuts, cookies, crisps, and the like. The math is simple: food-centric environment + debit or credit card = impulsive, live-to-regret-it food decisions.

Impulsive decisions to purchase pleasurable but unhealthy foods—a doughnut while purchasing coffee, our favorite chocolate bar when we stop at the store for milk and toilet paper—are based on spontaneous desires triggered by images and sensations. Such snap decisions, based on emotion rather than conscious thought, can undermine your long-term goals, such as sticking to a healthy eating plan.

So, in the age of debit cards, this is an old-school tool: if you're out and about and you want something to eat, pay cash only.

When it comes to impulse buys, it's all about the hard cash. From a psychological perspective, it's more "painful" to use cash than a credit card, which distances you from the experience and specifically the emotions directly connected to parting with cash, even a small amount. If you like to shop, you know that it's much harder to hand over a large amount of money than your credit card.

The same phenomenon applies to food purchases. In a six-month analysis of the shopping behaviors of a thousand people, published in the *Journal of Consumer Research,* researchers found that their carts held more foods rated as impulsive and unhealthy when credit or debit cards, rather than cash, were used to pay. In follow-up studies, they found that this was due to the "pain" of paying in cash.[6]

Given that you struggle so mightily to make healthy choices, understanding that using plastic increases your likelihood of buying unhealthy food may help you rein in impulse buys. My clients are often amazed when they try the following exercise, particularly those who are heavily reliant on their credit cards or have a company credit card. Even if they still purchase the doughnut or cookie, they notice that the process of using cash inserts an interesting mental pause that was not previously there. We need more of these mental pauses or mental shifts, breaks in the automatic nature of acting on our impulses.

Even if you don't use this exercise long-term, doing so for only a week will shift the way you think about buying food impulsively. You'll have experienced a natural pause—that little bit of psychological "pain" of parting with cash. This may be a new emotion for you and one that you'll remember and tap into when you need it.

1. The next time you go grocery shopping or out to dinner, leave your credit card at home. Set a reasonable amount that you want to spend and place this in your wallet, purse, or pocket. (I know it seems impossible, but many of my clients go directly to an ATM before they hit the supermarket or restaurant.)

2. Watch and marvel as you make wiser purchases and eating decisions. You have to; there's no choice. You need milk more than those chicken wings at the deli counter.

3. If you struggle with snacking at work, bring a limited amount of cash with you. If you have a trusted colleague, ask him or her to hold on to it for you. Each day, place any money that you don't spend on junk food or impulse buys in a jar. Use this later to buy something you really want—like new jeans.

If you already use cash and don't have a credit card, start to save your receipts of processed-food purchases. Add up how much you spend over the course of a week. It adds up quickly. Save that money in your jar too, and spend it on a non-food item that will give you pleasure.

Tool 23: Ordering Up Emotionally Intelligent Eating

Dining out is a part of life, even when you struggle with eating or weight. But there's reason for optimism—a recent study found that women who took part in a six-week meditative program called Mindful Restaurant Eating lost weight while dining out—without dieting.

In the study, published in the *Journal of Nutrition and Education Behavior*,[7] thirty-five women aged forty to fifty-nine, of varying weights, ate out at least three times a week. Of the participants, 30 percent were dieting. The researchers placed half the women in an "intervention group," which learned to do meditative exercises that involved focusing on the sight, smell, and texture of the food they ate to maximize enjoyment, as well as focusing on their hunger, satiety, and eating triggers. The remaining volunteers were placed in a control group.

All the women continued to eat at restaurants—six times a week, on average. Despite this, the women in the intervention group lost an average of 3.75 pounds and reduced their calorie intake by approximately 300 calories a day, which led to weight loss or management over time. The women in the control group didn't make any changes and thus didn't lose any weight or eat any differently. Although the program was tailored for restaurant dining, the researchers found that the women also consumed fewer calories at home as well.

While the study findings are preliminary, they echo what many of my clients tell me: they can still enjoy restaurant dining—and lose or manage weight—when they use mindful eating and EI skills. If this approach works for them, it will work for you!

For at least one week, commit to practicing all four parts of the following exercise. When you feel ready, begin using these skills at restaurants.

EXERCISE

SKILL: SELF-AWARENESS

Continuing to eat until you are "full" can be a recipe for overeating. Often, by the time you perceive you are full, you have already overeaten. In this exercise, you'll learn to become mindfully aware of the moment you are content and no longer hungry.

1. Before you eat your next meal at home, ask yourself how hungry you are—a little bit, a lot, or not at all.

2. After five bites, ask yourself the same question.

3. Repeat, taking five bites and asking the question, until you say, "Not hungry anymore and satisfied." This is your cue to put down your fork (or spoon).

4. Feel the difference between "full" and "satisfied." "Full" is often signaled by an expanding of your stomach, while "not hungry, but

satisfied" is signaled by the absence of hunger cues like a rumbling stomach or the absence of emptiness. It is also feeling content.

5. Continue to practice this skill at each meal until it comes naturally to you.

When you're ready, practice this skill at your favorite eatery. Remember, restaurant portions are huge, so you may reach the "not hungry, but satisfied" phase before your plate is empty. If that happens, ask your server for a box—and box up the leftovers right away.

SKILL: MINDING YOUR IMPULSES

When you're dining out, choosing your meal wisely is half the battle. A two-minute mindful pause between your first choice and your final choice can help you do just that.

Begin by noticing what is going on internally. If your inner voice is urgently speaking to you about what you want, you may suspect that your impulses are in play. If this is the case:

1. Before you go to the restaurant, see if its menu is posted online. If so, familiarize yourself with its healthy options and choose what you'll order now, when you have a cool head, rather than at the restaurant.

2. If the menu isn't posted online, go to the restaurant, open the menu, carefully review the options, and choose what you want. Then, close the menu for two minutes, pick it up again, and scan your options a second time. This time gap gives you the opportunity to think twice rather than order on impulse.

3. If your impulses usually win out or the decision is too fraught with emotion, think of one healthy meal that you like that you can generally find on any menu (for example, clear soup, a turkey burger with sautéed mushrooms, and a salad with balsamic vinaigrette dressing). Without opening the menu, use that meal as your default.

SKILL: ASSERTIVENESS

When you're dining out, requesting that your order be prepared a certain way (no cheese, please; no hash browns, thank you) can help you avoid overeating. And if hash browns appear on your plate anyway, you have the option of requesting that they be taken away so you won't eat them. But not everyone feels comfortable with making requests. If speaking up at a restaurant feels difficult to you, it can be helpful to "rehearse" at home.

1. Practice the following phrases (or whatever phrases ring true for you) aloud in front of a mirror.

    "I'd like the dressing on the side, please."

    "Could you please leave off the cream sauce? I would appreciate that."

    "I'd like to replace the fries with the grilled vegetables. Thank you for making that change!"

2. Repeat, adjusting your tone and pitch until they roll off your tongue.

3. Brainstorm some "tweaks" of your own. Repeat steps 1 and 2.

SKILL: "SEEING" MINDLESS EATING

As soon as you take your seat at a restaurant, size up what mindless over-eating would look like in this setting. Tune in. Consciously identify the food that pushes you from "content" to "overly full." It might be:

- one or two pieces of bread and butter (depends on the size of the bread)

- a serving of chips

- the cheese or large, oily croutons on your salad

- half of the starch on your plate (rice, or mashed potatoes with butter)

You might even consider moving these items to another plate to con-sciously remind you that these foods take you from "content" to "overly full."

Tool 24: Follow Your Nose

Emotionally intelligent people know themselves—and know which aromas affect their appetites. Knowing how the scent of food affects you can help you prepare for the moment you sniff out something you love. I'm thinking of hot doughnuts, fresh out of the fryer. Have you ever had a homemade doughnut, fresh from the fryer? Do you love them? (If you don't, conjure up an image of your favorite food—the one that plagues you with cravings.)

Okay, you're primed. Whether you envisioned that fresh, hot doughnut or some other treat, an image popped into your mind. It's also likely that you envisioned the smell of it—in the case of the doughnut, a rich and doughy scent.

Food cravings are part sight, part smell. That is, they are visual and olfactory in nature. Your mind imagines both the sight and scent of a particular food, and *poof!* The cravings intensify.

Not so long ago you would have been told to avoid thinking about doughnuts (weight-loss diet books tend to take this just-say-no approach). But recent research suggests a more powerful (and pleasurable) option: Distract your visual and olfactory modalities so they don't build a powerful image of the sight or smell of doughnuts. Your senses can take only so much input. You can fill up this channel with something besides food smells.

In a study of sixty-seven women, published in the journal *Appetite,* researchers in Australia compared the effects of food and non-food odors on chocolate cravings. One by one, the women—who'd been told not to eat or drink for two hours before the test—were led into a quiet room, placed in front of a computer monitor, and shown photo after photo of delectable chocolate foods and desserts, including chocolate cake, brownies, ice cream, and doughnuts. After viewing each photo, they were instructed to retain a mental image of the picture they'd just seen. Then they were given a whiff of one of three different odors—jasmine, green apple, or water (a neutral scent)—from vials held under their noses. (The researchers included water to ensure them that any craving-reducing effect was not caused by the act of sniffing.) Then the researchers asked their volunteers to rate their desire or urge for chocolate on a scale that ranged from no desire to extremely strong desire. The scent of jasmine reduced chocolate cravings far more effectively than the other scents, the researchers found.[8]

The nice thing about whiffing away cravings is the simplicity. One brief exposure to a scent has been shown to reduce cravings.[9] You don't have to hold a vial to your nose for longer than a few seconds.

If you happen to be a smoker, you might try this tool as part of your overall plan to quit smoking. A 1999 study of smokers found that smelling a pleasant odor, and at a later date an unpleasant one, reduced the craving for a cigarette compared to the neutral smell of water. (The study tested seven other scents—coconut, banana, peppermint, lemon, Vicks VapoSteam, vinegar, and floral.) While negative scents associated with memories were less helpful in quashing cravings, both positive and negative odors helped participants cope with cravings.[10]

EXERCISE

At a natural foods store, buy several small bottles of essential oil of jasmine or another scent you like. Keep one at work, one in the kitchen, and one in your purse. When you experience an intense craving for a particular food, take a whiff. The scent will help reduce or block the sensory images your imagination creates of the smell of a food you love, which ramps up cravings.

If you find that this tool works especially well for you, go one step further. Create a box of bottles of essential oils or tea candles of non-food scents that you can inhale when you experience a specific craving.

Tool 25: A Tool for the Chew-Happy

Do you simply like to chew, or do you often feel the urge to put something in your mouth even after a meal? Don't be embarrassed. I have plenty of clients who do. For them (and maybe for you), there's comfort in the sheer act of chewing. You may be surprised to learn that chewing helps regulate your emotions and rein in your impulses—key features of emotional intelligence.

To researchers, that comfort has a name: orosensory stimulation—the motion involved in satiation and the calming effect that comes from mouth movements. (Think of a baby nursing.) To almost everyone else, it's the satisfaction of crunching crisps or tearing into a thick slice of dense, chewy, crusty bread.

Of course, bread and crisps are part of the problem, but chewing gum may be part of the solution. For an activity frowned on by generations of school teachers, gum has a lot to offer if you struggle with food. Research suggests that the benefits are significant: reduced stress; improved mood; sharper, faster thinking;[11] and reduced hunger and cravings.[12] Even if you're not a chewing-gum fan, consider the benefits:

Reduces Stress. In a study conducted at Swinburne University in Australia, researchers divided forty people into two groups: those who chewed gum and those who didn't. Then they subjected both groups to a computerized test that had them perform a variety of cognitive tasks. The tasks simultaneously involved reaction time, selective attention (focus), and response inhibition (holding back a response)—a setup literally designed to induce heavy stress.[13]

Those who chewed gum while multitasking under these stressful conditions reported nearly 10 percent less anxiety during moderate stress compared to the non-chewers, the study found. At the same time, their alertness was 8 percent higher during moderate stress, compared to the non-chewers. They also had lower cortisol levels than the non-chewers, and their overall multitasking performance was a whopping 67 percent greater, compared to the non-chewers. The researchers didn't know why anxiety and performance were better, but this may involve improved blood flow in the brain.

Relaxes While Maintaining Alertness. Electroencephalography (EEG) studies have found that chewing gum produces brain-wave patterns similar to the brain state of people who are relaxed. At least one study suggests that the chewing may increase alpha waves—the brain waves associated with increased arousal.[14] It's thought that alpha waves create *relaxed concentration,* a feeling of both relaxation and alertness. What better state to be in when you're trying to decide what or how much to eat or to avoid boredom eating?

Helps Mental Processing. Researchers at St. Lawrence University in New York found that students performed better on cognitive tests when asked to chew gum. In fact, gum chewing increased alertness better than caffeine—

but only for fifteen to twenty minutes. The researchers attributed the short-term boost to what's called *mastication-induced arousal*. They mean that chewing is a physical activity that creates a physical response in readying the body for action.[15]

Enhances Cognitive Abilities. In one study, researchers divided eighty students into two groups—those who chewed gum five minutes before a series of tests and those who didn't. (The simple tests measured memory, verbal fluency, and other cognitive abilities.) The gum-chewing group tested better.[16] Another study found that chewing gum improved reaction times[17]—of benefit when you have to make a decision, such as what to order at a restaurant.[18] It's both the chewing and the flavor that can help perk you up.

Dulls Hunger and Appetite. Chewing gum for at least forty-five minutes significantly dulled hunger, appetite, and cravings for snacks, and promoted fullness, a study in the journal *Appetite* found. Researchers had fifty-three women come to their lab four different days for a standard lunch. Immediately afterward, the women rated their hunger, appetite, and cravings for sweet and salty snacks every hour for three hours. Then they came back to the lab later for a snack (either salty or sweet). Twice during this three-hour period, the women chewed gum for at least fifteen minutes on the hour for a total of forty-five minutes, and twice they did not. On two occasions salty snacks were provided, and on two occasions sweet snacks were provided. The researchers found that chewing gum before snacking reduced snack intake by about 10 percent and significantly dulled hunger and the desire to eat.[19]

A word of caution: Sometimes chewing gum works well—too well. It can turn from a tool to a compulsion. Keep it to a pack or less per day. And for the sake of your teeth, opt for sugarless.

EXERCISE

There's no step-by-step procedure for this tool, but if you'd like to try chewing gum to manage your moods and cravings, it's helpful to know when to pop a piece into your mouth. Most research has found that gum is most helpful when you begin to chew several minutes before you need the boost.[20] Here are some times to try it:

- as you peruse a menu, to promote a state of relaxed concentration, which can help you make insight-driven decisions

- when you're stressed, to release tension and avoid stress eating

- fifteen minutes before a meal, to reduce your appetite and increase your sense of fullness

- from three to fifteen minutes before you have to make a decision, to get that glucose pumping and improve your reaction time[21]

In addition to *when* to chew, for an extra burst of alertness, opt for peppermint gum. The scent of peppermint has been linked to increased alertness, some studies have found.

YOU'RE READY TO USE YOUR NEW FOOD SMARTS!

How do you feel? Confident? Nervous? A bit of both?

No matter *how* you feel, you've raised your Eat.Q., and it can only increase from here. As you learn to embrace and accept your feelings more fully, you'll gain more confidence in your ability to use those feelings to make eating decisions that benefit your health and well-being—conscious eating decisions based on your awareness and understanding of your feelings and the skills you can use to manage them. We're at the end of our journey together, but you're more than ready to strike out on your own!

In fact, you've accomplished more than you may realize. By working this plan, you've chosen to confront old hurts, embrace new ideas, and do something different rather than the same old thing (start another diet). Whether your goal is to lose weight or simply make peace with food, you're on your way!

I wish you well as you continue the journey. You've got everything you need to succeed. And while true change takes time, applied with patience, positivity, and commitment, the EAT method *can* make lasting and permanent changes to your eating habits. I know. I've seen it help my clients, and I believe it can work for you.

A few final words: Keep moving forward. Don't rest on your laurels, and don't shrink from an unshakable commitment to being true to yourself. As the great painter Pablo Picasso once said, "Action is the foundational key to all success." I believe that with all my heart. I also believe that such action stems from self-love. So, as you move forward, love yourself. Believe in yourself. Have hope. You'll be surprised at what you can achieve.

I've given you the tools, but the commitment and courage come from you. Dig deep and live mindfully. With time, you'll find that you've become a helper to someone else who struggles with food.

If you have questions, or want to share your success using the EAT method, I'd love to hear from you! Please feel free to drop me a line at drsusanalbers.com and eatq.com.

APPENDIX:
GREAT MOMENTS IN EI HISTORY

Interest in noncognitive intelligence (which taps into your ability to cope and respond well in social situations rather than remember facts and ace tests) goes back to Charles Darwin, the father of evolution, who suggested that survival hinges on understanding emotional expression (i.e., you feel fear, you run). Here are some of the milestones in the development of EI.

1920s: Edward Thorndike writes extensively on what he called "social intelligence."[1]

1955: David Wechsler develops the Wechsler Adult Intelligence Scale, which includes verbal and nonverbal types of intelligence—a significant departure from the traditional measure of IQ as a single entity.[2]

1983: Howard Gardner introduces the concept of multiple intelligences, identifying eight specific types: spatial, linguistic, logical-mathematical, bodily-kinesthetic, musical, interpersonal, intrapersonal, and naturalistic.[3]

1985: Clinical and organizational psychologist Dr. Reuven Bar-On creates the first measure of emotional and social intelligence, the EQ-i. His theory, which he began formulating in the early 1980s, is based on EQ (emotional quotient), which he coined in his early doctoral studies. Today, Bar-On continues to be active in publishing and research.[4]

1990: Dr. Peter Salovey of Yale University and Dr. John D. Mayer of the University of New Hampshire publish a landmark paper in the journal *Imagination, Cognition, and Personality.* The paper coins the term "emotional intelligence" and explains their four-branch theory of EI: perceiving emotions, using emotions to facilitate thinking, understanding emotional meanings, and managing emotions.[5] Today, Salovey and Mayer continue to be leading researchers in the field they pioneered; they have been joined by David Caruso, a management psychologist at Yale University.[6]

1995: Daniel Goleman's bestselling book *Emotional Intelligence* links EI to success and redefines how we assess intelligence and abilities.

Interest in EI continues today. Numerous articles on emotional intelligence can be found on eiconsortium.org. Also, many new books, like this one, show how to apply emotional intelligence to your daily life, such as *Search Inside Yourself* by Chade-Meng Tan, one of Google's earliest engineers. It's an engaging and insightful hybrid of EI and mindfulness. Not surprisingly, Daniel Goleman and Jon Kabat-Zinn, a renowned teacher of mindfulness, wrote the foreword for Tan's book.

ACKNOWLEDGMENTS

I can no other answer make, but, thanks, and thanks.

—William Shakespeare

I'd like to offer a sincere "thanks, and thanks" to the many people who made this book possible:

To my colleagues and the researchers cited in these pages, your groundwork has made this book (and my clinical work in my office) possible.

To all the pioneers of emotional intelligence, particularly Dr. Daniel Goleman, Dr. Peter Salovey, and Dr. John D. Mayer, your work has forever changed the way we view ourselves and the way we value the ability to connect and communicate with others.

To the many researchers, clinicians, and writers whose work I admire and respect, including Chade-Meng Tan, Dr. Jon Kabat-Zinn, Dr. Jean Kristeller, Dr. Kelly McGonigal, Dr. Barbara Rolls, Dr. Cynthia Bulik, Dr. Marion Nestle, Dr. Roy Baumeister, Dr. Janet Polivy, Dr. Elisha Goldstein, Dr. Lilian Cheung, Thich Nhat Hanh, Dr. Andrew Weil, Dr. David Ludwig, Dr. David Katz, Dr. Steven Stein, Ellen Langer, Evelyn Tribole, and Elyse Resch, you have all taught me a great deal about emotional intelligence, mindful eating, mindfulness, and healthy eating.

Thank you, Dr. Sara Gottfried, for contributing the inspiring foreword and for your thoughtful, motivational words of advice.

To Dr. Brian Wansink, your research and book *Mindless Eating* continues to inspire me to think about mindful and mindless eating in new ways. Your knack for practical and engaging research is a gift.

To the Cleveland Clinic, it has been a pleasure to be part of your professional staff for ten years!

To Nancy Hancock, for your fantastic editorial advice and support from the team of editors, copy editors, marketing, and publicity staff at HarperOne.

To the editors and colleagues who helped me launch my previous books— *Eating Mindfully; 50 Ways to Soothe Yourself Without Food; Eat, Drink & Be*

Mindful; and But I Deserve This Chocolate—although I have thanked you personally many times, I am still very grateful for your help transforming my work with mindful eating into print.

To Mark Bittman, Michael Pollan, Jenni Schaefer, Jennifer Weiner, Dr. Oz, Dr. Roizen, Geene Roth, and Marsha Hudnall at Green Mountain, your work inspires people to eat healthier. Each one of you writes about how we eat from a different but beneficial perspective—from the global to the personal.

To my clients, as always, I appreciate being a part of your life and the honor of being a part of your journeys.

To Celeste Fine, who has been everything one could wish for in an agent— hardworking, responsive, creative, and supportive. And to Sarah Cantin, you were instrumental in introducing me to Celeste.

To David Zyla, for your exceptional style advice; Peter James of Peter James Web Designs, for your exceptional web and technical assistance; and to Erika Harwood, for creating the beautiful graphics in this book.

To Julia VanTine, your hard work, persistence, and assistance helped me get each word just right.

To Carrie Arnold, for your research assistance and your own writing promoting healthy eating.

As always, a hug to my longtime friends—Dr. Victoria Gould, Jane Lesniewski , Betsy Swope, Eric Lingenfelter, and Dr. Jason Grief. I always look forward to spending time with you in various parts of the country. Many thanks to Susan Heady for reviewing my drafts many times and for your friendship.

To Dr. Thomas Albers, Carmela Albers, Dr. Angela Albers, Dr. Eric Brooks; Judd, Linda, Jenna, Paul, Maya, Jonah Serotta; and John, Rhonda, Jim Bowling, I know that I am extremely fortunate to have all of you—such a supportive family who are very involved and close by. Thank you to Angie for being ready to travel at a moment's notice—I look forward to many more adventures.

To John, Brooklyn, and Jack Bowling. Words can't express my appreciation of your support and partnership. Brookie and Jack—thank you for your daily words of wisdom and for the happiest of smiles.

NOTES

Chapter 1
The Solution to Emotional Eating, Stress Eating, and Plain Old Overeating

1. J. Brambila-Macias et al., "Policy Interventions to Promote Healthy Eating: A Review of What Works, What Does Not, and What Is Promising," *Food Nutrition Bulletin* 32, no. 4 (December 2011): 365–75, http://www.ncbi.nlm.nih.gov/pubmed/22590970.

2. Jon Kabat-Zinn, *Full Catastrophe Living: Using the Wisdom of Your Body and Mind to Face Stress, Pain, and Illness* (New York: Dell Publishing, 1991).

3. P. Salovey and J. D. Mayer, "Emotional Intelligence," *Imagination, Cognition, and Personality* 9, no. 3 (1990): 185–211, http://www.unh.edu/emotional_intelligence/EI%20 Assets/Reprints . . . EI%20Proper/EI1990%20Emotional%20Intelligence.pdf.

4. Salovey and Mayer, "Emotional Intelligence," 185–211.

5. The website of Daniel Goleman, accessed April 24, 2013, http://danielgoleman .info/biography/.

6. Daniel Goleman, "What Makes a Leader?" *Harvard Business Review,* January 2004, accessed April 18, 2013, http://hbr.org/2004/01/what-makes-a-leader/ar/1.

7. F. L. Brown and V. Slaughter, "Normal Body, Beautiful Body: Discrepant Perceptions Reveal a Pervasive 'Thin Ideal' from Childhood to Adulthood," *Body Image* 8, no. 2 (March 2011): 119–25, http://www.ncbi.nlm.nih.gov/pubmed/21419739.

8. P. C. Peter and D. Brinberg, "Learning Emotional Intelligence: An Exploratory Study in the Domain of Health," *Journal of Applied Social Psychology* 42, no. 6 (June 2012): 1394–414, http://onlinelibrary.wiley.com/doi/10.1111/j.1559-1816.2012.00904.x/abstract.

9. L. Zysberg and A. Rubanov, "Emotional Intelligence and Emotional Eating Patterns: A New Insight into the Antecedents of Eating Disorders?" *Journal of Nutrition Education and Behavior* 42, no. 5 (September–October 2010): 345–8, http://www.ncbi.nlm.nih.gov/pubmed/20637702.

Chapter 2
The Moment of Decision

1. Hans-Rüdiger Pfister and Gisela Böhm, "The Multiplicity of Emotions: A Framework of Emotional Functions in Decision Making," *Judgment and Decision Making* 3, no. 1 (January 2008): 5–17, http://www.sas.upenn.edu/~baron/journal/bb1.pdf.

2. K. J. Rotenberg and D. Flood, "Loneliness, Dysphoria, Dietary Restraint, and Eating Behavior," *International Journal of Eating Disorders* 25, no. 1 (January 1999): 55–64, http://www.ncbi.nlm.nih.gov/pubmed/9924653.

3. L. Brondel et al., "Acute Partial Sleep Deprivation Increases Food Intake in Healthy Men," *American Journal of Clinical Nutrition* 91, no. 6 (June 2010): 1550–9, http://www .ncbi.nlm.nih.gov/pubmed/20357041.

4. S. A. Turner et al., "Emotional and Uncontrolled Eating Styles and Chocolate Chip Cookie Consumption: A Controlled Trial of the Effects of Positive Mood Enhancement," *Appetite* 54, no. 1 (February 2010): 143–9, http://www.ncbi.nlm.nih .gov/pubmed/19815044.

5. T. Van Strien et al., "Emotional Eating and Food Intake After Sadness and Joy," *Appetite* 66 (July 2013): 20–5, http://www.ncbi.nlm.nih.gov/pubmed/23470231.

6. N. Rose et al., "Mood Food: Chocolate and Depressive Symptoms in a Cross-sectional Analysis," *Archives of Internal Medicine* 170, no. 8 (April 2010): 699–703, http:// www.ncbi.nlm.nih.gov/pubmed/20421555.

7. Brian Wansink and Jeffrey Sobal, "Mindless Eating: The 200 Daily Food Decisions We Overlook," *Environment and Behavior* 39, no. 1 (January 2007): 106–23.

8. Brandon Keim, "Brain Scanners Can See Your Decisions Before You Make Them," *Wired,* April 13, 2008, http://www.wired.com/science/discoveries/news/2008/04/mind_decision.

9. U. N. Danner et al., "Decision-Making Impairments in Women with Binge Eating Disorder in Comparison with Obese and Normal Weight Women," *European Eating Disorders Review* 20, no. 1 (January 2012): e56–62, http://www.ncbi.nlm.nih.gov/pubmed/21308871.

10. George Loewenstein, "Hot–Cold Empathy Gaps and Medical Decision Making," *Health Psychology* 24, no. 4 supplement (July 2005): S49–S56, https://www.rci.rutgers.edu/~gbc/psycDM/Loewenstein2005.pdf.

11. J. J. Arch and M. G. Craske, "Mechanisms of Mindfulness: Emotion Regulation Following a Focused Breathing Induction," *Behaviour Research and Therapy* 44, no. 12 (December 2006): 1849–58, http://www.ncbi.nlm.nih.gov/pubmed/16460668.

12. Arch and Craske, "Mechanisms of Mindfulness," 1849–58.

13. S. S. Iyengar and M. R. Lepper, "When Choice Is Demotivating: Can One Desire Too Much of a Good Thing?" *Journal of Personality and Social Psychology* 79, no. 6 (December 2000): 995–1006, http://www.columbia.edu/~ss957/articles/Choice_is_Demotivating.pdf.

14. E. M. Caruso and F. Gino, "Blind Ethics: Closing One's Eyes Polarizes Moral Judgments and Discourages Dishonest Behavior," *Cognition* 118, no. 2 (February 2011), 280–5, doi:10.1016/j.cognition.2010.11.008.

15. Barry Schwartz, *The Paradox of Choice: Why More Is Less* (New York: Ecco Press, 2003).

16. A. S. Hanks et al., "Healthy Convenience: Nudging Students Toward Healthier Choices in the Lunchroom," *Journal of Public Health* 34, no. 3 (August 2012): 370–6, doi:10.1093/pubmed/fds003.

Chapter 3
The EAT Method

1. K. Tapper et al., "Exploratory Randomised Controlled Trial of a Mindfulness-Based Weight-Loss Intervention for Women," *Appetite* 52, no. 2 (April 2009): 396–404, http://www.ncbi.nlm.nih.gov/pubmed/19101598.

2. Gayle M. Timmerman and Adama Brown, "The Effect of a Mindful Restaurant Eating Intervention on Weight Management in Women," *Journal of Nutrition Education and Behavior* 44, no. 1 (January–February 2012): 22–8, doi:10.1016/j.jneb.2011.03.143, http://www.jneb.org/article/S1499–4046(11)00264–8/fulltext.

3. A. J. Crum et al., "Mind Over Milkshakes: Mindsets, Not Just Nutrients, Determine Ghrelin Response," *Health Psychology* 30, no. 4 (July 2011): 424–9, http://www.ncbi.nlm.nih.gov/pubmed/21574706.

4. C. E. Cochrane et al., "Alexithymia in the Eating Disorders," *International Journal of Eating Disorders* 14, no. 2 (September 1993): 219–22, http://www.ncbi.nlm.nih.gov/pubmed/8401555.

5. B. M. Herbert et al., "Interoception Across Modalities: On the Relationship Between Cardiac Awareness and the Sensitivity for Gastric Functions," *PLOS ONE* 7, no. 5 (2012): e36646, http://www.plosone.org/article/info:doi/10.1371/journal.pone.0036646.

6. V. Ainley and M. Tsakiris, "Body Conscious? Interoceptive Awareness, Measured by Heartbeat Perception, Is Negatively Correlated with Self-Objectification," *PLOS ONE* 8, no. 2 (2013): e55568, http://www.plosone.org/article/authors/info%3Adoi%2F10.1371%2Fjournal.pone.0055568;jsessionid=789CFF5470F75A54BAA64050399A697C.

Chapter 4
Dieting

1. Karen Kaplan, "*Maggie Goes on a Diet* the Sensible Way in Children's Book," *Los Angeles Times,* August 23, 2011, http://articles.latimes.com/2011/aug/23/news/la-heb-maggie-goes-on-a-diet-book-20110823.

2. Bonnie Rochman, "*Maggie Goes on a Diet:* A Kids' Book About Dieting? Not Without Controversy," *Time,* August 25, 2011, http://healthland.time.com/2011/08/25/will-fat-kids-become-popular-if-they-go-on-a-diet-maggie-goes-on-a-diet-makes-the-case/.

3. N. R. Reyes et al., "Similarities and Differences Between Weight-Loss Maintainers and Regainers: A Qualitative Analysis," *Journal of the Academy of Nutrition and Dietetics* 112, no. 4 (April 2012): 499–505, http://www.ncbi.nlm.nih.gov/pubmed/22709701.

4. "McDonald's USA Nutrition Facts for Popular Menu Items," the website of the McDonald's Corporation, accessed April 15, 2013, http://nutrition.mcdonalds.com/getnutrition/nutritionfacts.pdf.

5. P. Rozin et al., "Operation of the Laws of Sympathetic Magic in Disgust and Other Domains," *Journal of Personality and Social Psychology* 50, no. 4 (1986): 703–12, http://www1.appstate.edu/~kms/classes/psy5150/Documents/RozinMagic86.pdf.

6. C. P. Herman, J. Polivy, and V. M. Esses, "The Illusion of Counter-Regulation," *Appetite* 9, no. 3 (December 1987): 161–9, http://www.ncbi.nlm.nih.gov/pubmed/3435133.

7. Jeni L. Burnette and Eli J. Finkel, "Buffering Against Weight Gain Following Dieting Setbacks: An Implicit Theory Intervention," *Journal of Experimental Social Psychology* 48, no. 3 (May 2012): 721–5, http://faculty.wcas.northwestern.edu/elifinkel/documents/2012_BurnetteFinkel_JESP.pdf.

8. Lawrence K. Altman, "Tarnower Was a Busy Physician, Too; Sportsman and Dinner Host a Veteran of World War II," *New York Times,* March 12, 1980, http://select.nytimes.com/gst/abstract.html?res=F00F16FE395C12728DDDAB0994DB405B8084 F1D3; Wolfgang Saxon, "Samm Sinclair Baker, 87, Author of Dozens of Self-Help Books," *New York Times,* March 23, 1997, http://www.nytimes.com/1997/03/23/nyregion/samm-sinclair-baker-87-author-of-dozens-of-self-help-books.html.

9. A. Massey and A. J. Hill, "Dieting and Food Craving: A Descriptive, Quasi-Prospective Study," *Appetite* 58, no. 3 (June 2012): 781–5, http://www.ncbi.nlm.nih.gov/pubmed/22306437.

10. E. M. Forman et al., "A Comparison of Acceptance- and Control-Based Strategies for Coping with Food Cravings: An Analog Study," *Behaviour Research and Therapy* 45, no. 10 (October 2007): 2372–86, doi:10.1016/j.brat.2007.04.004.

11. H. J. E. M. Alberts et al., "Coping with Food Cravings: Investigating the Potential of a Mindfulness-Based Intervention," *Appetite* 55, no. 1 (August 2010): 160–3, http://www.sciencedirect.com/science/article/pii/S019566631000365X.

12. Forman et al., "A Comparison," 2372–86.

13. A. Meule, C. Vögele, and A. Kübler, "Restrained Eating Is Related to Accelerated Reaction to High Caloric Foods and Cardiac Autonomic Dysregulation," *Appetite* 58, no. 2 (April 2012): 638-44, http://www.ncbi.nlm.nih.gov/pubmed/22142510.

14. Meredith Melnick, "The Cranky Dieter Explained: How Self-Control Makes You Angry," *Time,* March 22, 2011, http://healthland.time.com/2011/03/22/the-cranky-dieter-explained-self-control-makes-you-angry/.

15. "Nourish: Carbohydrates Fuel Your Brain," the website of the Franklin Institute, accessed April 15, 2013, http://www.fi.edu/learn/brain/carbs.html#brainenergy.

16. K. E. D'Anci et al., "Low-Carbohydrate Weight-Loss Diets: Effects on Cognition and Mood," *Appetite* 52, no. 1 (February 2009): 96–103, http://naldc.nal.usda.gov/download/23706/PDF.

17. E. Kemps, M. Tiggemann, and K. Marshall, "Relationship Between Dieting to Lose Weight and the Functioning of the Central Executive," *Appetite* 45, no. 3 (December 2005): 287–94, http://www.ncbi.nlm.nih.gov/pubmed/16126305/.

Chapter 5
Pleasure Seeking

1. Jean Anthelme Brillat-Savarin, *The Physiology of Taste: Or Meditations on Transcendental Gastronomy* (New York: Vintage, 2011).

2. Kent C. Berridge and Morten L. Kringelbach, "Affective Neuroscience of Pleasure: Reward in Humans and Animals," *Psychopharmacology* 199, no. 3 (August 2008): 457–80, http://www.lsa.umich.edu/psych/research&labs/berridge/publications/Berridge%20&%20Kringelbach%20Affective%20neuroscience%20of%20pleasure%20Psychopharmacology%202008.pdf.

3. Rush University Medical Center, "Obesity Counseling Should Focus on Neurobehavioral Processes, Not Personal Choice, Researchers Say," news release, August 1, 2011, http://www.rush.edu/webapps/MEDREL/servlet/NewsRelease?id=1514; B. M. Appelhans et al., "Time to Abandon the Notion of Personal Choice in Dietary Counseling for Obesity?" *Journal of the American Dietetic Association* 111, no. 8 (August 2011): 1130–6, http://www.ncbi.nlm.nih.gov/pmc/articles/PMC3148487/.

4. Berridge and Kringelbach, "Affective Neuroscience of Pleasure," 457–80.

5. Lauren Torrisi, "Sprinkles Installs Cupcake ATMs for 24-Hour Cravings," *ABC News*, March 2, 2012, http://abcnews.go.com/blogs/lifestyle/2012/03/sprinkles-installs-cupcake-atms-for-24-hour-cravings/.

6. Ozlem Ayduk et al., "Regulating the Interpersonal Self: Strategic Self-Regulation for Coping with Rejection Sensitivity," *Journal of Personality and Social Psychology* 79, no. 5 (2000): 776–92, http://www.ocf.berkeley.edu/~rascl/publications/ayduk_JPSP_2000.pdf.

7. T. R. Schlam et al., "Preschoolers' Delay of Gratification Predicts Their Body Mass 30 Years Later," *Journal of Pediatrics* 162, no. 1 (January 2013): 90–3, http://www.ncbi.nlm.nih.gov/pubmed/22906511.

8. Beatrice A. Golomb et al., "Association Between More Frequent Chocolate Consumption and Lower Body Mass Index," *Archives of Internal Medicine* 172, no. 6 (March 2012): 519–21, http://archinte.jamanetwork.com/article.aspx?articleid=1108800.

9. Harald Koegler, "Too Sweet to Be Real?" *Archives of Internal Medicine* 172, no. 16 (September 2012): 1270, http://www.ncbi.nlm.nih.gov/pubmed/22965392.

10. Beatrice A. Golomb, "'Too Sweet to Be Real?' Reply," Editor's Correspondence, The JAMA Network online, September 10, 2012, http://archinte.jamanetwork.com/article.aspx?articleid=1357453#References; Koegler, "Too Sweet to Be Real?," 1270.

11. M. Macht and J. Mueller, "Immediate Effects of Chocolate on Experimentally Induced Mood States," *Appetite* 49, no. 3 (November 2007): 667–74, http://www.ncbi.nlm.nih.gov/pubmed/17597253.

12. R. C. Havermans, "Stimulus Specificity but No Dishabituation of Sensory-Specific Satiety," *Appetite* 58, no. 3 (June 2012): 852–5, http://www.ncbi.nlm.nih.gov/pubmed/22343169.

13. Mary A. Gerend and Jon K. Maner, "Fear, Anger, Fruits, and Veggies: Interactive Effects of Emotion and Message Framing on Health Behavior," *Health Psychology* 30, no. 4 (July 2011), 420–3.

14. Harm Veling et al., "Using Stop Signals to Inhibit Chronic Dieters' Responses Toward Palatable Foods," *Behaviour Research and Therapy* 49 (2011): 771–80.

15. Justin Hepler et al., "Being Active and Impulsive: The Role of Goals for Action and Inaction in Self-Control," *Motivation and Emotion* 36, no. 4 (December 2012): 416–24, http://link.springer.com/article/10.1007%2Fs11031-011-9263-4.

16. A. E. Dingemans et al., "Expectations, Mood, and Eating Behavior in Binge Eating Disorder: Beware of the Bright Side," *Appetite* 53, no. 2 (October 2009): 166–73, http://www.ncbi.nlm.nih.gov/pubmed/19520125.

17. G. Parker, I. Parker, and H. Brotchie, "Mood State Effects of Chocolate," *Journal of Affective Disorders* 92, nos. 2–3 (June 2006): 149–59, http://www.ncbi.nlm.nih.gov/pubmed/16546266.

18. J. A. Erskine and G. J. Georgiou, "Effects of Thought Suppression on Eating Behaviour in Restrained and Non-restrained Eaters," *Appetite* 54, no. 3 (June 2010): 499–503, http://www.ncbi.nlm.nih.gov/pubmed/20152872.

Chapter 6
Social Eating

1. E. Robinson et al., "Social Matching of Food Intake and the Need for Social Acceptance," *Appetite* 56, no. 3 (June 2011): 747–52, http://www.ncbi.nlm.nih.gov/pubmed/21396972.

2. M. Kiernan et al., "Social Support for Healthy Behaviors: Scale Psychometrics and Prediction of Weight Loss Among Women in a Behavioral Program," *Obesity (Silver Spring)* 20, no. 4 (April 2012): 756–64, http://www.ncbi.nlm.nih.gov/pubmed/21996661.

3. M. A. Pachucki, P. F. Jacques, and N. A. Christakis, "Social Network Concordance in Food Choice Among Spouses, Friends, and Siblings," *American Journal of Public Health* 101, no. 11 (November 2011): 2170–7, http://christakis.med.harvard.edu/pdf/publications/articles/124.pdf.

4. Deborah Madison and Patrick McFarlin, *What We Eat When We Eat Alone* (Layton, UT: Gibbs Smith, 2009); "What We Really Eat When We Eat Alone," National Public Radio, July 5, 2009, http://www.npr.org/templates/story/story.php?storyId=106281310.

5. C. F. Bove, J. Sobal, and B. S. Rauschenbach, "Food Choices Among Newly Married Couples: Convergence, Conflict, Individualism, and Projects," *Appetite* 40, no. 1 (February 2003): 25–41, http://www.ncbi.nlm.nih.gov/pubmed/12631502.

6. R. C. J. Hermans et al., "Mimicry of Food Intake: The Dynamic Interplay Between Eating Companions," *PLOS ONE* 7, no. 2 (2012): e31027, http://www.ncbi.nlm.nih.gov/pmc/articles/PMC3270030/?tool=pubmed.

7. J. J. Exline et al., "People-Pleasing Through Eating: Sociotropy Predicts Greater Eating in Response to Perceived Social Pressure," *Journal of Social and Clinical Psychology* 31, no. 2 (2012): 169–93, http://guilfordjournals.com/doi/pdf/10.1521/jscp.2012.31.2.169.

8. J. D. Troisi and S. Gabriel, "Chicken Soup Really Is Good for the Soul," *Psychological Science* 22, no. 6 (June 2011): 747–53, http://pss.sagepub.com/content/22/6/747.

Chapter 7
Stress

1. "An Expert Opinion: Is There Really 'One Trick' to Losing Belly Fat," part 2, Rush University Medical Center online, http://www.rush.edu/rumc/page-1298330128627.html.

2. American Psychological Association, "Latest APA Survey Reveals Deepening Concerns About Connection Between Chronic Disease and Stress," press release, January 11, 2012, http://www.apa.org/news/press/releases/2012/01/chronic-disease.aspx.

3. United HealthCare Services, "The Stages of Stress," Stress newsletter, 2010, http://hr.columbus.gov/uploadedFiles/Human_Resources/Healthy_Columbus/Home/stress%20newsletter.pdf.

4. "How to Manage Stress," WebMD, 2009, http://www.webmd.com/balance/guide/all-stressed-out.

5. B. Foss and S. M. Dyrstad, "Stress in Obesity: Cause or Consequence?" *Medical Hypotheses* 77, no. 1 (July 2011): 7–10, http://www.ncbi.nlm.nih.gov/pubmed/21444159.

6. Foss and Dyrstad, "Stress in Obesity," 7–10.

7. "Is There Really 'One Trick,'" Rush University Medical Center online.

8. S. A. George et al., "CRH-Stimulated Cortisol Release and Food Intake in Healthy, Non-Obese Adults," *Psychoneuroendocrinology* 35, no. 4 (May 2010): 607–12, http://www.ncbi.nlm.nih.gov/pmc/articles/PMC2843773/.

9. Hara E. Marano, "Stress and Eating," *Psychology Today,* November 21, 2003, last

modified April 11, 2007, http://www.psychologytoday.com/articles/200311/stress-and-eating.

11. M. Smith, R. Segal, and J. Segal, "Stress Symptoms, Signs, and Causes," HelpGuide.org, last updated April 2013, http://helpguide.org/mental/stress_signs.htm.

12. Baba Shiv and Alexander Fedorikhin, "Heart and Mind in Conflict: The Interplay of Affect and Cognition in Consumer Decision Making," *Journal of Consumer Research* 26, no. 3 (December 1999): 278–92, http://www.mendeley.com/research/heart-mind-conflict-interplay-affect-cognition-consumer-decision-making-9/.

13. J. M. Born et al., "Acute Stress and Food-Related Reward Activation in the Brain During Food Choice During Eating in the Absence of Hunger," *International Journal of Obesity* 34, no. 1 (January 2010): 172–81, http://www.ncbi.nlm.nih.gov/pubmed/19844211.

14. U.S. Department of Agriculture, "Clementines Fact Sheet," May 11, 2013, http://healthymeals.nal.usda.gov/hsmrs/NJQuickSteps/NJ_Qk_Steps_Participant/Clementines.pdf.

15. U.S. Department of Agriculture, "Clementines Fact Sheet."

16. United HealthCare Services, "The Stages of Stress."

17. John Stossel and Frank Mastropolo, "Anger: Myths and Management," *20/20,* ABC News online, January 24, 2008, http://abcnews.go.com/2020/Stossel/story?id=4176825&page=1.

18. D. L. Katz et al., "Cocoa and Chocolate in Human Health and Disease," *Antioxidants and Redox Signaling* 15, no. 10 (November 15, 2011): 2779–811.

19. Elizabeth Somer, *Eat Your Way to Happiness* (New York: Harlequin, 2009), pp. 44–45.

20. M. A. Skinner et al., "Effects of Kiwifruit on Innate and Adaptive Immunity and Symptoms of Upper Respiratory Tract Infections," *Advances in Food and Nutrition Research* 68 (2013): 301–20, http://www.ncbi.nlm.nih.gov/pubmed/23394995.

21. L. Kass et al., "Effect of Magnesium Supplementation on Blood Pressure: A Meta-analysis," *European Journal of Clinical Nutrition* 66, no. 4 (April 2012): 411–18, http://www.ncbi.nlm.nih.gov/pubmed/22318649.

22. E. R. Bertone-Johnson et al., "Calcium and Vitamin D Intake and Risk of Incident Premenstrual Syndrome," *Archives of Internal Medicine* 165, no. 11 (June 13, 2005): 1246–52, http://www.ncbi.nlm.nih.gov/pubmed/15956003.

23. S. G. West et al., "Effects of Diets High in Walnuts and Flax Oil on Hemodynamic Responses to Stress and Vascular Endothelial Function," *Journal of the American College of Nutrition* 29, no. 6 (December 2010): 595–603, http://www.ncbi.nlm.nih.gov/pubmed/21677123.

24. A. Steptoe et al., "The Effects of Tea on Psychophysiological Stress Responsivity and Post-Stress Recovery: A Randomised Double-Blind Trial," *Psychopharmacology* (Berl) 190, no. 1 (January 2007): 81–89, http://www.ncbi.nlm.nih.gov/pubmed/17013636.

25. M. L. Dreher and A. J. Davenport, "Hass Avocado Composition and Potential Health Effects," *Critical Reviews in Food Science Nutrition* 53, no. 7 (2013): 738–50, http://www.ncbi.nlm.nih.gov/pubmed/23638933.

26. K. S. Kuehl, "Cherry Juice Targets Antioxidant Potential and Pain Relief," *Medicine and Sports Science* 59 (2012): 86–93, http://www.ncbi.nlm.nih.gov/pubmed/23075558.

27. M L. Dreher, "Pistachio Nuts: Composition and Potential Health Benefits," *Nutrition Reviews* 70, no. 4 (April 2012): 234–40, http://www.ncbi.nlm.nih.gov/pubmed/22458696.

Chapter 8
Trauma

1. J. K. Sandel, "The Effects of Trauma Exposure, Emotional Intelligence, and Positive Emotion on Resilience," *Dissertation Abstracts International Section B: The Sciences and Engineering* 69, no. 1-B (2008): 698, http://www.mendeley.com/research/effects-trauma-exposure-emotional-intelligence-positive-emotion-resilience-19/.

2. Mary Ellen Copeland, "Dealing with the Effects of Trauma: A Self-Help Guide," U.S. Department of Health and Human Services, Substance Abuse and Mental Health Services Administration, and the Center for Mental Health Services, http://store.samhsa.gov/shin/content/SMA-3717/SMA-3717.pdf.

3. "Post-Traumatic Stress Disorder," the website of the National Institute of Mental Health, last reviewed May 8, 2013, http://www.nimh.nih.gov/health/publications/post-traumatic-stress-disorder-ptsd/what-are-the-symptoms-of-ptsd.shtml.

4. "What Is Post-Traumatic Stress Disorder?," the website of the National Institute of Mental Health, last reviewed May 8, 2013, http://www.nimh.nih.gov/health/publications/post-traumatic-stress-disorder-ptsd/what-are-the-symptoms-of-ptsd.shtml.

5. "What Are the Symptons of Post-Traumatic Stress Disorder?," the website of the National Institute of Mental Health last reviewed May 8, 2013, http://www.nimh.nih.gov/health/publications/post-traumatic-stress-disorder-ptsd/what-are-the-symptoms-of-ptsd.shtml.

6. "Coping with Trauma," the website of Iona College, 2013, http://www.iona.edu/studentlife/counsel/guide/copingTrauma.cfm?.

7. Copeland, "Dealing with the Effects of Trauma.

8. S. L. Pagoto et al., "Association of Post-Traumatic Stress Disorder and Obesity in a Nationally Representative Sample," *Obesity* 20, no. 1 (January 2012): 200–5, http://www.ncbi.nlm.nih.gov/pubmed/22016096.

9. Pagoto et al., "Association of Post-Traumatic Stress Disorder and Obesity.

10. "What Are the Symptoms of PTSD?," the website of the National Center for PTSD, U.S. Department of Veterans Affairs, January 1, 2007, last modified March 26, 2013, http://www.ptsd.va.gov/public/pages/what-is-ptsd.asp.

11. "What Are the Symptoms of PTSD?," the website of the National Center for PTSD, U.S. Department of Veterans Affairs.

12. Erin Falconer et al., "The Neural Networks of Inhibitory Control in Posttraumatic Stress Disorder," *Journal of Psychiatry and Neuroscience* 33, no. 5 (September 2008): 413.

13. A. R. Armstrong, R. F. Galligan, and C. R. Critchley, "Emotional Intelligence and Psychological Resilience to Negative Life Events," *Personality and Individual Differences* 51, no. 3 (August 2011): 331–6.

Chapter 9
E: Embracing Your Feelings, Learning to Reconnect

1. Julie Steenhuysen (Reuters), "Name That Feeling: You'll Feel Better," *Lab News* (blog), Social Cognitive Neuroscience Laboratory, the website of the University of California, Los Angeles, June 20, 2007, http://www.scn.ucla.edu/AL/sciam.html.

2. University of California, Los Angeles, "Putting Feelings into Words Produces Therapeutic Effects in the Brain," news release, *ScienceDaily* online, June 22, 2007, http://www.sciencedaily.com/releases/2007/06/070622090727.htm.

3. B. Wansink, J. M. Painter, and K. Van Ittersum, "Descriptive Menu Labels' Effect on Sales," *Cornell Hotel and Restaurant Administrative Quarterly* 42, no. 6 (December 2001): 68–72, http://foodpsychology.cornell.edu/research/summary-descriptive-labels.html.

4. Iris W. Hung and Aparna A. Labroo, "From Firm Muscles to Firm Willpower:

Understanding the Role of Embodied Cognition in Self-Regulation," *Journal of Consumer Research* 37, no. 6 (April 2011): 1046–64.

5. Samuel McNerney, "A Brief Guide to Embodied Cognition: Why You Are Not Your Brain," *Scientific American Guest Blog*, November 4, 2011, http://blogs.scientificamerican.com/guest-blog/2011/11/04/a-brief-guide-to-embodied-cognition-why-you-are-not-your-brain/.

6. G. Finlayson, N. King, and J. Blundell, "The Role of Implicit Wanting in Relation to Explicit Liking and Wanting for Food: Implications for Appetite Control," *Appetite* 50, no. 1 (January 2008): 120–7, http://www.ncbi.nlm.nih.gov/pubmed/17655972.

7. A. J. Brown, L. T. Smith, and L. W. Craighead, "Appetite Awareness as a Mediator in an Eating Disorders Preventions Program," *Eating Disorders* 18, no. 4 (July 2010): 286–301, http://www.ncbi.nlm.nih.gov/pubmed/20603730.

Chapter 10
A: Accepting Your Emotions, Understanding Their Meaning

1. M. Hoerger et al., "Emotional Intelligence: A Theoretical Framework for Individual Differences in Affective Forecasting," *Emotion* 12, no. 4 (August 2012): 716–25, http://www.ncbi.nlm.nih.gov/pmc/articles/PMC3330168/.

2. B. Q. Ford and M. Tamir, "When Getting Angry Is Smart: Emotional Preferences and Emotional Intelligence," *Emotion* 12, no. 4 (August 2012): 685–9, http://www.ncbi.nlm.nih.gov/pubmed/22309721.

3. P. Lally et al., "How Habits Are Formed," *European Journal of Social Psychology* 40, no. 6 (October 2010): 998–1009, http://onlinelibrary.wiley.com/doi/10.1002/ejsp.674/abstract;jsessionid=D3A517310AD3DD8943E0E6E56A29898C.d03t01.

4. Marla Paul (Northwestern University), "Less Couch Time Equals Fewer Cookies," news release, *ScienceDaily* online, May 28, 2012, http://www.sciencedaily.com/releases/2012/05/120528175627.htm.

5. P. M. Ullrich and S. K. Lutgendorf, "Journaling About Stressful Events: Effects of Cognitive Processing and Emotional Expression," *Annals of Behavioral Medicine* 24, no. 3 (Summer 2002): 244–50, http://www.scopus.com/record/display.url?eid=2-s2.0-0036022094&origin=inward&txGid=3AtXTO_hmHEeFkKHWO0M4PH%3a2.

6. Bonnie A. White et al., "Many Apples a Day Keep the Blues Away—Daily Experiences of Negative and Positive Affect and Food Consumption in Young Adults," *British Journal of Health Psychology* (January 24, 2013), http://www.ncbi.nlm.nih.gov/pubmed/23347122.

Chapter 11
T: Turning to New, Positive Alternatives to Eating

1. K. A. Page et al., "Circulating Glucose Levels Modulate Neural Control of Desire for High-Calorie Foods in Humans," *Journal of Clinical Investigation* 121, no. 10 (October 2011): 4161–9, http://www.ncbi.nlm.nih.gov/pmc/articles/PMC3195474/.

2. David Gal and Wendy Liu, "Grapes of Wrath: The Angry Effects of Self-Control," *Journal of Consumer Research* 38, no. 3 (2011): 445–58.

3. A. Meule, J. Westenhöfer, and A. Kübler, "Food Cravings Mediate the Relationship Between Rigid, but Not Flexible Control of Eating Behavior and Dieting Success," *Appetite* 57, no. 3 (December 2011): 582–4, http://www.ncbi.nlm.nih.gov/pubmed/21824503.

4. J. Andrade et al., "Use of a Clay Modeling Task to Reduce Chocolate Craving," *Appetite* 58, no. 3 (June 2012): 955–63, http://www.ncbi.nlm.nih.gov/pubmed/22369958.

5. J. L. Burnette and E. J. Finkel, "Buffering Against Weight Gain Following Dieting Setbacks: An Implicit Theory Intervention," *Journal of Experimental Social Psychology* 48, no. 3 (May 2012): 721–5, http://faculty.wcas.northwestern.edu/eli-finkel/documents/2012_BurnetteFinkel_JESP.pdf.

6. M. Thomas, K. K. Desai, and S. Seenivasan, "How Credit Card Payments Increase

Unhealthy Food Purchases: Visceral Regulation of Vices," *Journal of Consumer Research* 38, no. 1 (June 2011): 126–39, http://www.jcr-admin.org/files/press PDFs/101810122129_thomas-visceralrevulationofvices.pdf.

7. Gayle M. Timmerman and Adama Brown, "The Effect of a Mindful Restaurant Eating Intervention on Weight Management in Women," *Journal of Nutrition Education and Behavior* 44, no. 1 (Jan–Feb 2012): 22–8, doi:10.1016/j.jneb.2011.03.143, http://www.jneb.org/article/S1499–4046(11)00264–8/fulltext.

8. E. Kemps, M. Tiggemann, and S. Bettany, "Non-Food Odorants Reduce Chocolate Cravings," *Appetite* 58, no. 3 (June 2012): 1087–90, http://www.ncbi.nlm.nih.gov/pubmed/22407134.

9. E. Kemps and M. Tiggemann, "Olfactory Stimulation Curbs Food Cravings," *Addictive Behaviors* 38, no. 2 (February 2013): 1550–4, http://www.ncbi.nlm.nih.gov/pubmed/22766488.

10. M. A. Sayette and D. J. Parrott, "Effects of Olfactory Stimuli on Urge Reduction in Smokers," *Experimental and Clinical Psychopharmacology* 7, no. 2 (May 1999): 151–9, http://www.ncbi.nlm.nih.gov/pubmed/10340155.

11. Andrew P. Smith, "Effects of Chewing Gum on Cognitive Function, Mood, and Physiology in Stressed and Non-Stressed Volunteers," *Nutritional Neuroscience* 13, no. 1 (February 2010): 7–16, http://www.ncbi.nlm.nih.gov/pubmed/20132649.

12. M. M. Hetherington and M. F. Regan, "Effects of Chewing Gum on Short-Term Appetite Regulation in Moderately Restrained Eaters," *Appetite* 57, no. 2 (October 2011): 475–82, http://www.ncbi.nlm.nih.gov/pubmed/21718732.

13. A. Scholey et al., "Chewing Gum Alleviates Negative Mood and Reduces Cortisol During Acute Laboratory Psychological Stress," *Physiology and Behavior* 97, nos. 3–4 (June 2009): 304–12, http://www.ncbi.nlm.nih.gov/pubmed/19268676.

14. A. P. Smith, K. Chaplin, and E. Wadsworth, "Chewing Gum, Occupational Stress, Work Performance, and Well-Being: An Intervention Study," *Appetite* 58, no. 3 (June 2012): 1083–6, http://www.sciencedirect.com/science/article/pii/S0195666312000943.

15. S. V. Onyper et al., "Cognitive Advantages of Chewing Gum: Now You See Them, Now You Don't," *Appetite* 57, no. 2 (October 2011): 321–8, http://www.ncbi.nlm.nih.gov/pubmed/21645566.

16. Onyper et al., "Cognitive Advantages of Chewing Gum," 321–8.

17. Smith, "Effects of Chewing Gum," 7–16.

18. Smith, "Effects of Chewing Gum," 7–16.

19. Hetherington and Regan, "Effects of Chewing Gum," 475–82.

20. Onyper et al., "Cognitive Advantages of Chewing Gum," 321–8.

21. Onyper et al., "Cognitive Advantages of Chewing Gum," 321–8.

Appendix
Great Moments in EI History

1. R. L. Thorndike and S. Stein, "An Evaluation of the Attempts to Measure Social Intelligence," *Psychological Bulletin* 34, no. 5 (May 1937): 275–85, http://journals.ohiolink.edu/ejc/article.cgi?issn=00332909&issue=v34i0005&article=275 aeotatmsi.

2. David Wechsler, "Non-Intellective Factors in General Intelligence," *Psychological Bulletin* 37 (1940): 444–5, http://journals.ohiolink.edu/ejc/article.cgi?issn=0096851x&issue=v38i0001&article=101_nfigi.

3. Howard Gardner, *Frames of Mind: The Theory of Multiple Intelligences,* 3rd ed. (New York: Basic Books, 2011).

4. Reuven Bar-On, "The Development of a Concept of Psychological Well-Being," unpublished doctoral dissertation, Rhodes University, South Africa (1988), http://connection.ebscohost.com/c/articles/48480770/emotional-intelligence-integral-part-positive-psychology.

5. Salovey and Mayer, "Emotional Intelligence," 185–211.

6. J. D. Mayer, D. R. Caruso, and P. Salovey, "Emotional Intelligence Meets Traditional Standards for an Intelligence," *Intelligence* 27, no. 4 (December 1999): 267–98.

INDEX